Plant-Based Diet

Clean Eating Is Important

Kenneth A. Dunmire

Copyright ©2022 by Chasity T. Overman

All rights reserved.

No portion of this book may be reproduced in any form without written permission from the publisher or author, except as permitted by U.S. copyright law.

Contents

1. INTRODUCTION — 1
2. A PLANT-BASED DIET'S CHARACTERISTICS — 40
3. ADD DIETARY SUPPLEMENTS ON A DAILY BASIS OR IN CYCLES — 62
4. Onions with peppers Masala — 78
5. Onions with a sweet and sour taste — 96
6. Himalayan salt with black pepper — 114
7. Chickpea Salad is a salad made with chickpeas — 131

Chapter 1

INTRODUCTION

Beginner's Guide to a Plant-Based Diet

A Life Philosophy. Clean Eating Is Important For Long-Term Health. Delicious Chocolate Desserts and a 14-Day Detox Meal Plan are among the special recipes.

Author : Chasity T. Overman

In recent years, the plant-based diet has become one of the most popular searches on Google.

It's a contentious diet among "conventional dietitians" since it doesn't precisely adhere to the World Health Organization's nutritional requirements.

It is undeniable that diet-related issues have always piqued the interest of a sizable portion of the global population.

It's also true that, despite recent improvements in economic well-being, we're dealing with a generation of individuals who are sick from a young age. We only include food intolerances, pollen allergies, medicine allergies, powder allergies, and food sensitivities; however, we should consider how much the number of fat or overweight individuals has risen in the previous fifty years, as well as the prevalence of autoimmune, cancer, and heart disease.

We are individuals who have improved our life expectancy on average, but at 40-50 years of age, we begin to take medicine that will be with us for the rest of our lives.

At some point, individuals begin to ask themselves questions, and they may begin to wonder whether their sicknesses and burdening of their bodies are not caused by what they consume.

The solution to these questions might be a plant-based diet.

A crucial concept must not be overlooked: the human body's vital energy and its ability to cure itself.

A PLANT-BASED DIET'S CHARACTERISTICS

A way of life philosophy

The vegetable-based diet has been one of the most popular eating fads for quite some time now.

This diet is more of a philosophy of life than a basic diet, based on the idea that food is not just "fuel" for the body, but also "care" for it.

Food and mental and physical well-being have a very intimate, almost inseparable link.

Mind. An antidote to the unpleasant feelings we've become used to, such as worry, panic, and despair, is a well-balanced, clean diet.

Proper nutrition aids in regaining emotional control.

Body. You may restore control of your metabolism and weight when you reclaim control of your body.

The major goal of this diet is to cleanse and restore fresh vitality to the body and mind, allowing us to enhance our current health.

It's important to remember that enhancing our current health involves safeguarding our future health.

This diet combines plant-based macronutrients (carbohydrates, proteins, and fats) with plant-based micronutrients (vitamins, minerals, and fibers).

Foods that are high in preservatives, refined, industrially processed, or canned are not permitted.

Because it is based on foods that are "vibrant with vitality" and "pure from industrial pollution," this diet is referred to as "electric-alkalizing."

Furthermore, this kind of diet has a powerful anti-inflammatory effect due to the body's thorough cleansing.

BEGINNER'S GUIDE TO A PLANT-BASED DIET

In two devoted chapters of this book, the characteristics of the alkalizing and anti-inflammatory diet will be discussed.

A wise decision

There's no doubting that health and nutrition are inextricably linked. Food is the finest medication you can take.

We may make a significant contribution to our health by eating the proper foods, just as we can create the optimum circumstances for illness to develop by eating the wrong foods.

A large body of scientific evidence now supports the health advantages that a vegetable-based diet may provide.

According to the American Dietetic Association, a well balanced plant-based diet is nutritious, nutritionally sufficient, and provides health advantages in the prevention and treatment of many illnesses.

Even the most omnivorous of diets should contain a large amount of plant-based meals.

A diet rich in fruits, vegetables, legumes, whole grains, and low in salt, sugar, and alcohol is recommended for the prevention of chronic degenerative disorders.

These foods, which are high in polyphenols, vitamins, and minerals, have the ability to reduce inflammation, alkalize our systems, and boost our immunological defenses.

Vegetarian foods also include a lot of fiber, which helps to properly support the gut flora.

change the bacteria in your gut from putrefactive to fermentative

Toxic metabolites must be removed from the organism.

We'll go through the link between a plant-based diet, alkaline pH, inflammation, and the immune system in more detail later.

Veganism's beginnings in history

Veganism may be characterized as a plant-based diet.

Many people assume that veganism is a relatively new concept, yet it really began in 1847 in Ramsgate, England, with the foundation of the Vegetarian Society, the world's oldest vegetarian organization. This organization was split into two groups in the early 1920s: those who favoured a vegetarian diet and those who refused to use dairy products and other animal-derived derivatives.

The Vegan Society and the name Vegan were formed as a consequence of combining some of the first three letters of the word "Vegetarian" with the final two letters of the word "Vegetarian."

Vegan thought grew swiftly in 1945, with the publication "The Vegan" already having 500 subscribers. It managed to promote a new understanding connected not just to food but also to numerous concerns relating to the environment, animal rights, and social coexistence.

A true cultural revolution, a shift in how we view everything around us, a true philosophy that has managed to include natural medicine, agriculture, and nutrition studies in a very short period of time.

In 1970, this movement sparked interest in "official" medicine to the point that it prompted the launch of new research, particularly in the United States, which led to the demonization of diets high in animal fats and proteins, which were labeled as damaging to one's health.

In 2010, a considerable portion of the world's population embraced the vegan ideology, and this was aided by the increased availability of formerly difficult-to-find food supplies.

I'm not going to debate the merits of which diets are more or less "ethical." This is not the book's intention.

People who choose to be vegan do so not simply for moral reasons, but also because they believe that only a certain sort of vegan cuisine will prevent people from being unwell, or even cure them if they are already ill.

In general, I believe that a diet must be long-term sustainable, and that it must be a pleasurable habit that stems from a deliberate decision. To put it another way, the way we eat must become a part of who we are and how we live.

Whatever your dietary preferences are, whether or not they prohibit animal products, a plant-based diet has shown to be a viable option as a detox plan to be followed once or twice a year, for example, for two weeks every three to four months.

After the recipes, there is a full 14-day food plan at the conclusion of the book.

An anti-inflammatory diet is one that consists of foods that are low in inflammation.

Inflammation seems to be one of the most efficient methods for the body to react to diverse external and internal stimuli, according to the most current evolutionary theories.

Even a little wound might not heal without a strong inflammatory response.

Inflammation, like stress, must be an emergency reaction that is equally beneficial in the short term as it is harmful if it is active all of the time.

Inflammation becomes the source of many contemporary pathologies such as cardiovascular illnesses, hypertension, diabetes, dementia, obesity, cancers, autoimmune disorders, and so on when it develops a permanent and systemic condition.

As reported in the venerable journal "Science," "One of the most significant discoveries in medicine in the past two decades is the discovery of inflammation as the pathophysiological process that causes all chronic illnesses.

The majority of the population has a hidden inflammation that goes unnoticed and seems to be innocuous.

A diet high in lactose, gluten, omega 6 (found in sunflower oil and most foods processed by the food industry), and sweets stimulates the start of a latent inflammation that will eventually become chronic.

Obesity produces inflammation, which creates a vicious cycle in which inflammation makes losing weight more difficult. Overweight will be discussed in a different chapter.

Numerous research conducted throughout the globe have attempted to define the nutrients that must be included in an anti-inflammatory diet. Take, for example, a major research published in 2010 in the Nutrition Journal that looked at the antioxidants in 3100 commonly consumed foods throughout the globe.

In conclusion, while designing an anti-inflammatory diet, keep in mind that it will not be a single meal or supplement that will be helpful, but rather the synergy of foods that contain diverse antioxidant molecules to prevent inflammation.

The following is an example of an anti-inflammatory eating plan based on the studies cited above:

5 servings of high-antioxidant fruits and vegetables (berries, red plums, spinach, broccoli, etc.); 2 servings of hot beverages such as herbal teas 1 citrus fruit, squeezed; vegetable oils, such as extra virgin olive oil; Nuts and avocados are high in omega 3 fatty acids.

A plant-based diet is alkaline.

An alkaline diet is a healthy diet that tries to keep our body's acid-base balance in check.

The pH permits us to maintain our body's acid-base balance by representing it as a numerical number.

On a scale of 1 to 14, PH is calculated (we are talking about acid PH for values below 7 and basic PH for higher values). After digestion, test the pH of the meals to determine which are acidic and which are alkaline. Assuming that the PH level in our circulation is somewhat acidic, alkaline meals should be prioritized in order to maintain a healthy acid-base balance.

Can food be classified as acidic or alkaline based on what principles?

The ash that remains after the meal has been digested is tested to determine the basic acid content of the food.

It's vital to note that there are meals that are classed as acidic but are turned into alkaline based after a sequence of chemical events that trigger digestion. This is how it usually works in healthy people. The Potential Renal Acid Load, often known as the PRAL index, is the most well-known metric for determining a food's PH level. This index categorizes foods into two groups:

PRAL + meals have an acidifying impact (such as dairy products, fish, eggs, meat and fish).

PRAL-containing meals are alkalizing (fruits and vegetables).

An alkaline diet, which is popular in alternative medicine, prioritizes basic foods (also known as "alkaline"), such as diverse vegetables and fruits, which should be consumed raw whenever possible to preserve the vast amounts of fundamental minerals they contain (calcium, magnesium and potassium).

Due to their ability to restore the intestinal flora, scientific investigations have proven that alkaline meals are helpful to both our metabolism and the health of our gut.

If we want to dramatically reduce our body's acidity level, we may perform alkaline fasting, which is an extreme variant of this diet. Only alkaline meals should be consumed in this instance, and only water and herbal infusions should be consumed as liquids. Some dietitians, however, warn against continuing this technique in the long run since it may result in significant nutritional deficits.

How critical is our body's acid-base balance?

Now we're getting close to understanding why so many people opt to eat an alkaline diet. The explanation is simple: our acid-base balance is affected by this diet. As a result, those who follow this diet will avoid achieving dangerously high levels of acidity in their bodies.

But, precisely, what does "acid-base balance" imply?

It's the body's connection between acidity and alkalinity in a nutshell.

In truth, our bodies are equipped with a mechanism known as the "buffer system," which attempts to maintain the body's proper acid-base balance, avoiding harmful imbalances and changes in acidity and alkalinity.

However, if we eat a diet high in acidic foods, the buffer mechanism may become ineffective, resulting in hyperacidity.

Various symptoms and disorders, such as weariness, digestive issues, migraines, muscular or joint difficulties, might emerge in this situation.

So, although our buffer system is self-contained, it must not be overworked and, at the very least, it must be regenerated on a regular basis.

A diet that boosts your immune system

The immune system is the body's first line of defense against pathogens, acting as a rapid response mechanism. As a result, having a weakened immune system exposes you to more diseases and infections.

The intestine is primarily responsible for influencing this defense mechanism: it is estimated that the intestine contains 80 percent of the immune system's cells.

The microbiota is made up of entire colonies of microorganisms that live inside the intestine. A healthy microbiota keeps us safe from the dangerous and latent general inflammatory state that puts us at risk of becoming ill.

Several studies have shown how an alkaline and anti-inflammatory diet, such as a paint-based diet, affects our immune system's strength and efficiency.

What micronutrients must be present in our diet in order for our immune systems to function properly?

Fatty acids: Fatty acids are the cell's outer layer's supporting structure. In order to enter and multiply, viruses require a host cell. As a result, a diet rich in healthy fatty acids, such as those found in avocado, dried fruits, olive oil, and other vegetable-based oils, helps to strengthen the outer layer of cells, making it more difficult for viruses to enter.

Antioxidants are molecules that aid in the defense of the organism against harmful agents and the state of oxidative stress.

Which is the most crucial?

Glutathione is a substance produced by our bodies and found in a variety of foods such as avocado, spinach, peaches, and apples. Then there are foods that stimulate Glutathione production, such as garlic, onion, red fruits and vegetables, which are high in Selenium.

Vitamin C is found in high concentrations in all green vegetables, berries, and citrus fruits; because it has a higher bioavailability, it is best to get this vitamin from fresh foods rather than supplements.

Vitamin D deficiency is directly linked to an ineffective immune system; recent surveys have revealed that over 70% of the world's population is vitamin D deficient. It's abundant in vegetables, particularly mushrooms.

Carrots, pumpkin, parsley, ripe tomatoes, broccoli, and green cabbage are high in B-carotene (a precursor to Vitamin A) "..

Other micronutrients useful for keeping the immune system efficient and ready to react to external "aggressions" include selenium, zinc, and copper, which are found in legumes, mushrooms, and almonds and are important metals for their antioxidant activity.

Because they are high in fiber, probiotics and prebiotics found in all fruits and vegetables keep the microbiota healthy.

As you may have noticed, these are the same ingredients that make up the foundation of an alkaline and anti-inflammatory diet.

IT'S EASY TO INCLUDE A PLANT-BASED DIET IN YOUR LIFESTYLE.

How to properly balance your meals throughout the day

It's simple because a plant-based diet is diverse and abundant in foods that give the nutrients the body needs to operate optimally:

Fibers such as whole grains, which are preferable if naturally gluten-free, proteins mostly from legumes, healthy fats derived from dried fruit, vitamins and minerals from nature's numerous fruits and vegetables

In 2014, the Vegan Plate was published in the Journal of the Academy of Nutrition and Dietetics, a very helpful tool that helps you to correctly organize your plant nutrition in order to consume all of the nutrients essential to keep us healthy. With over 25000 members, this nutritionist organization is one of the biggest and most prominent in the world. Anyone may download the article for free.

The Vegan Plate is a fantastic visual depiction based only on plant meals that may maintain the proper balance of all the vital nutritional components that our bodies need. Fruits, vegetables, nuts, oilseeds, lipids, and proteins are the six primary dietary categories that include these vital components.

We placed nutritional ingredients high in vitamin B12 and vitamin D in the middle of the plate to underline the relevance of these two vitamins in a well balanced plant diet. It is crucial to begin by calculating one's daily calorie needs. These needs vary based on whether you are a man or a woman, the sort of employment you do, and the amount of physical activity you engage in.

Once the daily calorie needs have been calculated, the vegan plate may simply be split into the six food groups listed above.

So, instead of using scales or calorie computations to figure out what to put on your plate, just follow the vegan plate's easy and helpful guidelines.

To properly distribute meals throughout the day, they should be divided into three major meals with one or two snacks in between.

Breakfast like a king, lunch like a middle-class person, and supper like a poor, according to an ancient adage.

Breakfast should consist of a decent herbal tea, vegetable milk, or coffee. If you like, you may add bitter cocoa or dark chocolate crumbles to a porridge made with whole cereal flakes, vegetarian yogurt, dried fruit, and chia seeds. A fruit may be eaten to round out your morning.

Fruit, such as berries with low fructose content, or dried fruit, slices of dry coconut, or high-quality dark chocolate chips, should be included in snacks.

Lunch and supper should contain a substantial number of vegetables, ideally fresh but also cooked or merely blanched, in order to provide the necessary nutrients. You will be able to receive all of the required enzymes to better tackle digestion if you start your meal with vegetables; also, since vegetables have a satiating capacity, you will be more likely to finish the meal without caloric excesses. Lunch may also be followed with a meal made with gluten-free cereals, particularly whole wheat, or a dish made with vegetable proteins such those found in legumes.

The following is a list of gluten-free cereals or gluten-free cereals that include a particularly digestible kind of gluten, such as spelt:

Amaranth

rice that is black in color

Kamut

Quinoa

Rya

Emmer

Rice that has been harvested from the wild

During the day, herbal teas brewed with the plants listed below are recommended:

Raspberry red Alvaca Clove Chamomille Anice Fennel Ginger

Tea made with sea moss

Lemongrass

Using spices as an ingredient in all of one's foods is also highly advised. The following is a list of healthful spices with descriptions of their properties:

Curcumin is an antioxidant that benefits brain, cardiovascular, and joint health. Dandelion is a blood and liver purifier.

Elderberry (Sambucus nigra) - helps to protect the body against colds. Burdock root is a blood and liver cleanser that also acts as a diuretic.

Vitamin and mineral supplements made from bladderwrack (seaweed). Bromelain and papain are enzymes that break down proteins in the small intestine.

Proteins, vitamins and minerals, and detoxifiers are all found in chlorella (seaweed). Vitamin and mineral supplements made from Irish moss (seaweed).

Antiviral oregano oil

Blood cleanser, antibacterial, anti-inflammatory, and diuretic sarsaparilla Parasite-killing wormwood leaf

Vitamin and mineral supplements made from kelp (seaweed).

Flaxseed - rich essential fatty acids, prevents heart disease, cancer, and diabetes

Breakfast ideas that are both healthy and delicious

Cappuccino with soy milk

Two pieces of whole wheat spelt bread with a spread of creamy dried fruit like hazelnuts, almonds, or pistachios, as well as thin slices of fresh fruit like bananas

a cup of espresso

A cup of white vegetable yogurt topped with cereal flakes, chopped almonds, and sliced fresh fruit. Flax or chia seeds, which are high in omega 3 fatty acids, may be sprinkled on top.

Lunch as an example

Pitas with chickpea hummus, olives, and green leafy veggies on top. These veggies are exceptionally high in calcium, allowing individuals who follow a plant-based diet to meet their calcium needs without ingesting dairy products.

Apple slices with cinnamon and almond cream on top.

Dinner as an example

Quinoa with cooked peas and finely sliced zucchini

Avocado and walnut salad with flax seed oil dressing.

Sport and a plant-based diet

Sporting exercise is beneficial for more than simply weight loss and body sculpting. It's first and foremost a health-related decision.

To perform effective sports activity, we must understand how to feed our bodies with "clean" meals that give us with the required energy and aid in the recovery of our bodies after we have participated in sports.

Many well-known athletes, such as Carl Lewis, have shown that a plant-based diet may help them attain high levels of athletic performance.

Those who consume a vegetable-based diet do well in sports and, more importantly, recover rapidly after engaging in physical exercise.

The lactic acid produced by the body adds to the feeling of exhaustion experienced while participating in sports.

Because the tissues are already alkaline, the body creates less lactic acid while eating a plant-based diet, and the lactic acid created by the body under stress is "buffered" and disposed of more rapidly.

Plant foods having a high protein content, such as beans, are recommended for athletes. The legumes with the greatest protein are:

soybeans

beans in a wide sense

lupins

Even among cereals, those with a greater protein content are preferable:

oats

amaranth\sspelt

quinoa\sbuckwheat

Finally, oilseeds and dried fruits have a high protein content: There are a few that are particularly high in protein: linseeds, pumpkin seeds

seeds of sesame

pinecones

almonds

Spirulina, which is high in protein and iron, is the most well-known "doping" for athletes who consume veggies.

So, there are a few secrets to improving athletic performance: all you have to do is know them!

HOW TO EMPOWER YOURSELF WITH A PLANT-BASED DIET

Step one: INCLUDE THOSE FOODS IN YOUR DAILY DIET THAT HAVE BEEN CLASSIFIED AS SUPERFOODS BY THE MEDICAL-SCIENTIFIC LITERATURE.

Avocado is a powerhouse of beneficial nutrients. It's high in potassium and magnesium, mineral salts that play a role in all cellular interactions; it's also high in fiber and fatty acids. Our bodies can simply employ the latter to make energy, avoiding insulin surges that contribute to body fat buildup. Avocado has been found in recent research to be effective in preventing cancer, particularly stomach and pancreatic cancer, combating osteoporosis, and reducing the symptoms of depression.

Blueberries and red fruits are high in antioxidants, which reduce cellular aging. They also have a purifying and anti-inflammatory activity, which helps decrease blood sugar levels, and they encourage the rise of good HDL cholesterol, which strengthens the whole cardiovascular system. Despite their low sugar content, they are a concentrated source of taste that should not be overlooked in smoothies or salads....

Cumin: A spice with a strong scent that originates from the seeds of a herbaceous plant; high in calcium, magnesium, phosphorus, vitamin A, and vitamin E; good for boosting the immune system and keeping harmful viruses at bay.

Cinnamon: Known for its aphrodisiac effect and ability to enhance flavors in the kitchen for more than 2000 years; rich in phenols that slow down the putrefaction of certain foods; regulates cholesterol levels, facilitates digestion, reduces blood glucose levels, enhances energy, and even has mood-boosting properties.

Cabbage and broccoli: Crucifers are cold-tolerant and high in antioxidants like vitamin K, vitamin A, vitamin E, magnesium, omega 3 fibers, iron, and potassium; a 100-gram serving of broccoli contains 150 percent of our daily vitamin C requirement; medical literature recognizes these plants as having strong anti-carcinogenic properties; they prevent diseases like diabetes and osteoporosis, fortify the immune system, and promote weaning. Raw or pan-seared is preferable.

Coconut oil is derived from the coconut fruit. Rich in MCT medium-chain triglycerides, which are more easily used by our bodies to produce energy than fats from animals, which are defined as long-chain; as a result, when you eat coconut, its fat is immediately oxidized by the liver, providing energy; as a result, it is very suitable for those who practice sports;

however, it is also suitable for those who want to lose weight because, on the one hand, it prevents body fat accumulation and, on the other hand, it

Because of the lauric acid in it, it has significant antibacterial, viral, and fungal properties.

Turmeric is an antioxidant spice with potent anti-oxidant and anti-cancer properties, and it is widely used in holistic and ayurvedic medicine. Curcumin, the key component, has anti-inflammatory properties and is used to treat arthritis, inflammation, arthrosis, and joint discomfort. Turmeric also has the ability to protect the immune system.

Chocolate: It must include a high proportion of cocoa, at least 80%, and be raw if possible. It is recommended that you eat no more than 30 grams of sugar every day.

The term "food of gods" is used to describe chocolate. It's abundant in:

Antioxidants in magnesium

Tryptophan is a vital amino acid that helps to calm the nervous system and enhance the quality of sleep. It also contains polyphenols, which help to boost brain function and decrease cognitive decline. Blood pressure and cholesterol are controlled by flavonoids, which preserve the interior wall of blood vessels.

You'll discover some delicious chocolate-based desserts in the recipes section!

Step two: ADD DIETARY SUPPLEMENTS ON A DAILY BASIS OR IN CYCLES.

It may be useful to augment the plaint based diet with various dietary supplements to enhance the favorable benefits.

Vitamin B-12 (cobalamin)

Vitamin B-12 is required for the proper functioning of blood and brain cells, as well as the creation of DNA.

People who eat a vegan or vegetarian diet, as well as those who are older, are at risk of acquiring B-12 deficiency.

Fatigue, depression, tingling in the hands and feet, and anemia are all symptoms of B-12 insufficiency.

Essential Fatty Acids Omega-3

Omega-3 essential fatty acids are essentially made up of the different components of cell membranes. They are beneficial in the following areas:

sustaining healthy heart health and a good cardio circulatory system brain functioning and visual health energy

Vitamin C, often known as ascorbic acid, is a water-soluble vitamin.

Although a plant-based diet is abundant in vitamin-rich foods, it is still necessary to include this vitamin since today's agricultural soils are less fertile than those of the past, and as a result, fruits may not contain as much vitamin C as they formerly did.

We're also talking about a vitamin that is rapidly degraded by heat, so we aren't always able to absorb it in the proper amounts.

Because it is involved in so many metabolic and enzymatic activities, it is one of the most essential vitamins:

Strengthens immunological defenses, improving immune cells' capacity to create antibodies and hence the body's ability to better withstand all illnesses.

It aids in the detoxification of the body (toxins resulting from smoke or pollution).

By altering collagen formation, it protects and restores tissues; the latter protects the functions of cartilage, bones, skin, capillaries, and gums.

It is an antioxidant because it counteracts the detrimental effects of free radicals, or chemicals that promote premature aging in our bodies.

It is beneficial in the event of anemia because it enhances iron digestion, which is a crucial mineral for the synthesis of red blood cells.

It reduces stress by assisting in the creation of chemicals that maintain nerve impulse transmission steady, as well as regulating the manufacture of the stress hormone.

Vitamin D is an important nutrient.

Our bodies can only create vitamin D when they are exposed to sunlight.

It may be beneficial to include this vitamin in one's diet if they are infrequently exposed to the sun or just during specific seasons of the year.

This vitamin is vital for the following reasons:

Because it aids in maintaining an appropriate level of calico in the blood, it is necessary for proper mineralization of bones and teeth.

To support the health of our kidneys, arteries, and bodily tissues; to improve the immune system against illnesses and viruses

Maintaining the heart's and cardio-circulatory system's functioning.

Step three: CHOOSE HIGH-QUALITY FOOD AND AVOID GENETICALLY MODIFIED FOOD.

Because this is a detox diet, it's preferable to choose organic or sustainable bio food that's free of chemicals and heavy metals to maximum efficacy.

Step four is to:

DRINK A LOT OF WATER, PREFERABLY SPRING WATER.

Drinking lots of water every day is crucial since water is necessary for a healthy and efficient body; also, water aids in nutrient absorption.

Drinking spring water would be excellent.

Water that runs from rocks or deep soils is known as spring water, and it is a dynamic, active, and vital element.

As a result, spring water has a rich and pleasant flavor. It hydrates and refreshes us better than tap water or other forms of water.

If the source is alpine, the water is filtered by earthy and sandy layers that work as a filter, preventing heavy contaminants from entering the water; as a result, we are dealing with waters that are normally quite pure.

It's also referred to as 'dynamized water,' which is water that has the power to energize the body's cells while also being beneficial to the excretory organs like the kidneys and liver.

When purchasing spring water, ensure sure the source's name and location, as well as a statement of bottling at the source, are put on the bottle label.

FOOD: THE ORIGINAL ANTI-DISEASE MEDICINE

Weight loss with a plant-based diet

We've seen how a plant-based diet may improve health by preventing and curing major illnesses.

Is it, however, causing you to lose weight?

When it comes to losing weight, even this sort of diet must adhere to the concept of calorie deficit: no deficit, no weight loss. While it isn't a diet's credo, it is the "hidden" idea at the heart of all weight-loss diets.

Weight reduction is a natural result of following a plant-based diet since the foods it comprises are often low in calories and satiating due to their high water and dietary fiber content.

The accumulation of body fat, particularly in the belly, is a precursor to the onset of various illnesses such as diabetes, autoimmune disorders, and oncological diseases.

As a result, it's critical not to dismiss this early signal from the body and to act quickly to get the metabolic system back on track.

To this purpose, a plant-based diet is beneficial since it has many fibers that have a satiating and fulfilling impact, allowing us to go longer without feeling hungry; it also contains little saturated fats.

Neurodegenerative illness and a plant-based diet

Food is made up of chemical and biological molecules that interact with our cells, including neurons, and may have a positive or negative influence depending on the quality of the food we consume.

Neurons are unable to replicate and regenerate if all cells reproduce and renew. They have the ability to rejuvenate but not reproduce. As a result, it is preferable to safeguard them as much as possible, particularly after they reach a certain age.

Mercury, lead, and other environmentally hazardous ions accumulate specifically in adipose tissue and nerve tissue with a fat component.

Chronic inflammation may contribute to the beginning and progression of neurodegenerative disorders like Alzheimer's and dementia, which are becoming more common: the central nervous system is composed up of neurons that, when inflamed, cause the nervous system to malfunction.

The good news is that nature always provides us with solutions. We may opt to consume "The Magnificent Seven," a group of entirely vegetarian meals that nourish and maintain the central nervous system.

Let's practice using them all on a daily basis:

Green tea tastes better when had first thing in the morning.

When ginger and turmeric are used as fresh roots, they are more effective.

Dark chocolate tastes better when it is processed raw, which implies that the cocoa beans used to make chocolate must not have been heated over 42 degrees.

Berries are high in vitamins, minerals, and polyphenols and provide a lot of them.

Dried fruits, with the exception of peanuts, which are allergenic and inflammatory. Walnuts are chosen because their form resembles that of our brain. They are anti-inflammatory and high in omega 3.

Flax seeds, chia seeds, and hemp seeds are all good sources of omega-3 fatty acids.

Chlorella tea is a freshwater alga that has powerful cleansing properties.

Conclusion

Maintaining a diet over time and keeping it sustainable seems to be far more difficult than getting started on one. While most individuals stick to a diet for a short amount of time, until they achieve their objectives, converting the diet into a new eating regimen to include into their lifestyle is exceedingly challenging.

A tactic called as "crowding out" is one approach to persuade us to eat healthier meals. It's simple: instead of removing unhealthy items from your diet, you can just incorporate better ones. Consider the following scenario:

You can gradually incorporate new healthy eating habits: the more often you eat healthy meals, the more likely you are to become accustomed to them and eventually prefer them to harmful ones; you can start the meal with a certain amount of raw vegetables: this will increase satiety and alkalize the meal; you can gradually incorporate new healthy eating habits: the more often you eat healthy meals, the more likely you are to become accustomed to them and eventually start preferring them to harmful ones. It only takes a few weeks to form a new habit; it is preferable to go shopping when you are not hungry: When we buy food when we aren't hungry, we make impulsive choices that aren't particularly reasonable; keep in mind that choosing veggie food is an ethical and environmentally sustainable decision.

If our health is excellent or if we already have diseases, switching to a plant-based diet can only bring one thing if we place ourselves in the best possible situation: the ability to heal ourselves. benefits. It's important to realize that our bodies are quite powerful.

Numerous scientific studies have shown that a healthy diet may prevent various ailments and, in many instances, cure them till they go away completely.

However, many individuals are unwilling to prioritize a healthy lifestyle in their everyday lives. People who suffer from chronic diseases are often those who consume foods that inflame their bodies on a regular basis, don't commit enough time to exercise, and live in constant tension, unable to cleanse their bad thoughts with a few minutes of meditation or deep relaxation each day.

In a future book, I'd want to go through all of these issues in more depth.

For the time being, I was content to share what I had learned about clean, green, anti-inflammatory, and healing diet with you.

I genuinely hope I was able to demonstrate how much we can improve the quality of our lives by just "consuming" what we have selected with conscience and knowledge, rather than what is easily accessible.

Continued success on your own path toward a more "conscious" diet!

RECIPES The following recipes are a collection of simple to make meals that show that healthy eating can be delicious as well.

And now, good luck with your meal!

Lasagna with carasau bread – cover picture – Preparation time: 20 minutes

Time to prepare: 20 minutes

4 servings

Ingredients:

200 g pita bread or carasau bread Soy milk (700 mL)

almond flour (40 g) spinach, 400 g

spelt flour (70 g) Nutmeg, salt, and pepper

olive oil (extra virgin)

Preparation:

Boil the spinach, then remove it from the water and set it aside to cool.

In a separate saucepan, whisk together the flour and soy milk until well combined.

Season to taste with salt, pepper, and nutmeg.

Bring the béchamel sauce to a low boil, stirring constantly, until it becomes creamy. Allow time for cooling.

Add the spinach and two tablespoons of oil.

Form the layers of lasagna in a casserole dish by alternating the spinach cream with carasau bread that has been gently wet with a little water or soy milk. Add the almond flour in between each layer.

Serve with a piece of corasau bread on the side. Place in a preheated oven at 200 degrees for 20 minutes after adding a little oil.

Nutrition

350 calories per serving fat (4 g)

Carbohydrates: 59 g Protein: 19 g

Tartare with avocado, tofu, and asparagus

The preparation time is 20 minutes.

Time to cook: 10 minutes

2 servings

Ingredients:

250 grams of asparagus

Tofu, sliced into cubes, 80 g a single lime

4 tbsp olive oil (extra virgin) 40 pine nuts, lightly roasted

a pinch of mustard powder seasoning with salt and pepper

garlic powder, a sprinkle basil leaves

Preparation:

Cook for 10 minutes with the asparagus.

Oil, garlic, half a lime juice, basil, and mustard powder should all be emulsified together.

To keep the avocado from darkening, dice it and sprinkle the remaining lime juice over it.

In a large mixing bowl, toss the chopped asparagus, avocado, and tofu with the oil emulsion.

Pour half of the compost into a ramekin that has been put in the middle of the dish to make the tartare.

Toasted pine nuts may be used as a garnish.

Nutrition

A serving has 440 calories and 35 grams of fat. Carbohydrates: 5,9 g Protein: 18 g

Crackers made with flaxseed

The preparation time is 20 minutes. Time to cook: 10 minutes

6 servings Ingredients:

200 g flour (millet or spelt) a teaspoon of dried chives 35 g extra virgin olive oil

Flax seeds, 60 g a teaspoon of salt and 200 mL of water

Preparation:

In a large mixing basin, combine all of the ingredients and mix with your hands until you have a homogenous dough.

Form the dough into a ball, cover it in plastic wrap, and place it in the refrigerator for two hours.

Preheat the oven to 200 degrees Fahrenheit.

On baking paper, roll out the dough into a rectangle with a relatively thin thickness.

Place the dough on an oven dish and cut it into cracker-sized pieces using a knife.

Preheat the oven to 350°F and bake for 10 minutes.

Remove the crackers from the oven and set them aside to cool before separating them.

Nutrition

195 calories per serving Fat content: 11 g Carbohydrates: 20 g Protein: 11 g

Casserole of Cabbage Rolls with a Twist

The preparation time is 10 minutes.

Time to cook: 40 minutes

4 servings

Ingredients:

1 cup quinoa (cooked) a red onion and a half

2 garlic cloves, finely chopped four white mushrooms, minced

one and a half cans diced tomatoes, finely chopped 8 green cabbage leaves, whole teaspoons of extra virgin olive oil, vegetable stock or homemade vegetable broth cup of fresh basil leaves, minced

Instructions:

Preheat the oven to 350 degrees Fahrenheit (180 degrees Celsius).

In a non-stick pan, combine the extra virgin olive oil, onion, quinoa, garlic clove, and sliced mushrooms. 5 minutes in the oven Combine the tomato sauce, vegetable stock, and basil in a mixing bowl. Mix thoroughly. Cook for a further ten minutes.

2 cabbage leaves should be placed on top of the baking sheet. Place a quarter of the filling on top of the cabbage leaves and tie them together with kitchen twine. Make the next three rolls in the same manner.

Cover with aluminum foil and bake in the oven for 40 minutes.

Before serving, allow for a 10-minute resting time.

Nutrition

261 calories per serving fat (2 g)

Carbohydrates: 51 g Protein: 12 g

Mango, Quinoa, and Black Bean Casserole with a Tangy Sauce

The preparation time is 10 minutes.

Time to prepare: 25 minutes

4 servings

Ingredients:

coconut milk (two cups)

2 cups cooked quinoa 1 cup vegetable stock or homemade vegetable broth

Rinse and drain 2 cups black beans, rinsed and ready to use 1/4 cup fresh mint (minced) mango, peeled and chopped 1 peeled and chopped avocado

a pinch of pink Himalayan salt

extra virgin olive oil (teaspoons)

Instructions:

Preheat the oven to 425 degrees Fahrenheit (200 degrees Celsius).

In a casserole dish, combine the stock, milk, and quinoa and stir thoroughly.

Cover with aluminum foil and bake for 25 minutes.

Remove the baking dish from the oven and turn it off. In a large mixing bowl, combine the beans, mango, avocado, and fresh mint.

Season with salt and olive oil before serving.

Nutrition

A serving has 573 calories. fat (23 g) Carbohydrates: 75 g protein (15 g)

Chapter 2

A PLANT-BASED DIET'S CHARACTERISTICS

A way of life philosophy

The vegetable-based diet has been one of the most popular eating fads for quite some time now.

This diet is more of a philosophy of life than a basic diet, based on the idea that food is not just "fuel" for the body, but also "care" for it.

Food and mental and physical well-being have a very intimate, almost inseparable link.

Mind. An antidote to the unpleasant feelings we've become used to, such as worry, panic, and despair, is a well-balanced, clean diet.

Proper nutrition aids in regaining emotional control.

Body. You may restore control of your metabolism and weight when you reclaim control of your body.

The major goal of this diet is to cleanse and restore fresh vitality to the body and mind, allowing us to enhance our current health.

It's important to remember that enhancing our current health involves safeguarding our future health.

This diet combines plant-based macronutrients (carbohydrates, proteins, and fats) with plant-based micronutrients (vitamins, minerals, and fibers).

Foods that are high in preservatives, refined, industrially processed, or canned are not permitted.

Because it is based on foods that are "vibrant with vitality" and "pure from industrial pollution," this diet is referred to as "electric-alkalizing."

Furthermore, this kind of diet has a powerful anti-inflammatory effect due to the body's thorough cleansing.

In two devoted chapters of this book, the characteristics of the alkalizing and anti-inflammatory diet will be discussed.

A wise decision

There's no doubting that health and nutrition are inextricably linked. Food is the finest medication you can take.

We may make a significant contribution to our health by eating the proper foods, just as we can create the optimum circumstances for illness to develop by eating the wrong foods.

A large body of scientific evidence now supports the health advantages that a vegetable-based diet may provide.

According to the American Dietetic Association, a well balanced plant-based diet is nutritious, nutritionally sufficient, and provides health advantages in the prevention and treatment of many illnesses.

Even the most omnivorous of diets should contain a large amount of plant-based meals.

A diet rich in fruits, vegetables, legumes, whole grains, and low in salt, sugar, and alcohol is recommended for the prevention of chronic degenerative disorders.

These foods, which are high in polyphenols, vitamins, and minerals, have the ability to reduce inflammation, alkalize our systems, and boost our immunological defenses.

Vegetarian foods also include a lot of fiber, which helps to properly support the gut flora.

change the bacteria in your gut from putrefactive to fermentative

Toxic metabolites must be removed from the organism.

We'll go through the link between a plant-based diet, alkaline pH, inflammation, and the immune system in more detail later.

Veganism's beginnings in history

Veganism may be characterized as a plant-based diet.

Many people assume that veganism is a relatively new concept, yet it really began in 1847 in Ramsgate, England, with the foundation of the Vegetarian Society, the world's oldest vegetarian organization. This organization was split into two groups in the early 1920s: those who favoured a vegetarian diet and those who refused to use dairy products and other animal-derived derivatives.

The Vegan Society and the name Vegan were formed as a consequence of combining some of the first three letters of the word "Vegetarian" with the final two letters of the word "Vegetarian."

Vegan thought grew swiftly in 1945, with the publication "The Vegan" already having 500 subscribers. It managed to promote a new understanding connected not just to food but also to numerous concerns relating to the environment, animal rights, and social coexistence.

A true cultural revolution, a shift in how we view everything around us, a true philosophy that has managed to include natural medicine, agriculture, and nutrition studies in a very short period of time.

In 1970, this movement sparked interest in "official" medicine to the point that it prompted the launch of new research, particularly in the United States, which led to the demonization of diets high in animal fats and proteins, which were labeled as damaging to one's health.

In 2010, a considerable portion of the world's population embraced the vegan ideology, and this was aided by the increased availability of formerly difficult-to-find food supplies.

I'm not going to debate the merits of which diets are more or less "ethical." This is not the book's intention.

People who choose to be vegan do so not simply for moral reasons, but also because they believe that only a certain sort of vegan cuisine will prevent people from being unwell, or even cure them if they are already ill.

In general, I believe that a diet must be long-term sustainable, and that it must be a pleasurable habit that stems from a deliberate decision. To put it another way, the way we eat must become a part of who we are and how we live.

Whatever your dietary preferences are, whether or not they prohibit animal products, a plant-based diet has shown to be a viable option as a detox plan to be followed once or twice a year, for example, for two weeks every three to four months.

After the recipes, there is a full 14-day food plan at the conclusion of the book.

An anti-inflammatory diet is one that consists of foods that are low in inflammation.

Inflammation seems to be one of the most efficient methods for the body to react to diverse external and internal stimuli, according to the most current evolutionary theories.

Even a little wound might not heal without a strong inflammatory response.

Inflammation, like stress, must be an emergency reaction that is equally beneficial in the short term as it is harmful if it is active all of the time.

Inflammation becomes the source of many contemporary pathologies such as cardiovascular illnesses, hypertension, diabetes, dementia, obesity, cancers, autoimmune disorders, and so on when it develops a permanent and systemic condition.

As reported in the venerable journal "Science," "One of the most significant discoveries in medicine in the past two decades is the discovery of inflammation as the pathophysiological process that causes all chronic illnesses.

The majority of the population has a hidden inflammation that goes unnoticed and seems to be innocuous.

A diet high in lactose, gluten, omega 6 (found in sunflower oil and most foods processed by the food industry), and sweets stimulates the start of a latent inflammation that will eventually become chronic.

Obesity produces inflammation, which creates a vicious cycle in which inflammation makes losing weight more difficult. Overweight will be discussed in a different chapter.

Numerous research conducted throughout the globe have attempted to define the nutrients that must be included in an anti-inflammatory diet. Take, for example, a major research published in 2010 in the Nutrition Journal that looked at the antioxidants in 3100 commonly consumed foods throughout the globe.

In conclusion, while designing an anti-inflammatory diet, keep in mind that it will not be a single meal or supplement that will be helpful, but rather the synergy of foods that contain diverse antioxidant molecules to prevent inflammation.

The following is an example of an anti-inflammatory eating plan based on the studies cited above:

5 servings of high-antioxidant fruits and vegetables (berries, red plums, spinach, broccoli, etc.); 2 servings of hot beverages such as herbal teas 1 citrus fruit, squeezed; vegetable oils,

such as extra virgin olive oil; Nuts and avocados are high in omega 3 fatty acids.

A plant-based diet is alkaline.

An alkaline diet is a healthy diet that tries to keep our body's acid-base balance in check.

The pH permits us to maintain our body's acid-base balance by representing it as a numerical number.

On a scale of 1 to 14, PH is calculated (we are talking about acid PH for values below 7 and basic PH for higher values). After digestion, test the pH of the meals to determine which are acidic and which are alkaline. Assuming that the PH level in our circulation is somewhat acidic, alkaline meals should be prioritized in order to maintain a healthy acid-base balance.

Can food be classified as acidic or alkaline based on what principles?

The ash that remains after the meal has been digested is tested to determine the basic acid content of the food.

It's vital to note that there are meals that are classed as acidic but are turned into alkaline based after a sequence of chemical events that trigger digestion. This is how it usually works in healthy people. The Potential Renal Acid Load, often known as the PRAL index, is the most well-known metric for determining a food's PH level. This index categorizes foods into two groups:

PRAL + meals have an acidifying impact (such as dairy products, fish, eggs, meat and fish).

PRAL-containing meals are alkalizing (fruits and vegetables).

An alkaline diet, which is popular in alternative medicine, prioritizes basic foods (also known as "alkaline"), such as diverse vegetables and fruits, which should be consumed raw whenever possible to preserve the vast amounts of fundamental minerals they contain (calcium, magnesium and potassium).

Due to their ability to restore the intestinal flora, scientific investigations have proven that alkaline meals are helpful to both our metabolism and the health of our gut.

If we want to dramatically reduce our body's acidity level, we may perform alkaline fasting, which is an extreme variant of this diet. Only alkaline meals should be consumed in this instance, and only water and herbal infusions should be consumed as liquids. Some dietitians, however, warn against continuing this technique in the long run since it may result in significant nutritional deficits.

How critical is our body's acid-base balance?

Now we're getting close to understanding why so many people opt to eat an alkaline diet. The explanation is simple: our acid-base balance is affected by this diet. As a result, those who follow this diet will avoid achieving dangerously high levels of acidity in their bodies.

But, precisely, what does "acid-base balance" imply?

It's the body's connection between acidity and alkalinity in a nutshell.

In truth, our bodies are equipped with a mechanism known as the "buffer system," which attempts to maintain the body's proper acid-base balance, avoiding harmful imbalances and changes in acidity and alkalinity.

However, if we eat a diet high in acidic foods, the buffer mechanism may become ineffective, resulting in hyperacidity.

Various symptoms and disorders, such as weariness, digestive issues, migraines, muscular or joint difficulties, might emerge in this situation.

So, although our buffer system is self-contained, it must not be overworked and, at the very least, it must be regenerated on a regular basis.

A diet that boosts your immune system

The immune system is the body's first line of defense against pathogens, acting as a rapid response mechanism. As a result, having a weakened immune system exposes you to more diseases and infections.

The intestine is primarily responsible for influencing this defense mechanism: it is estimated that the intestine contains 80 percent of the immune system's cells.

The microbiota is made up of entire colonies of microorganisms that live inside the intestine. A healthy microbiota keeps us safe from the dangerous and latent general inflammatory state that puts us at risk of becoming ill.

Several studies have shown how an alkaline and anti-inflammatory diet, such as a paint-based diet, affects our immune system's strength and efficiency.

What micronutrients must be present in our diet in order for our immune systems to function properly?

Fatty acids: Fatty acids are the cell's outer layer's supporting structure. In order to enter and multiply, viruses require a host cell. As a result, a diet rich in healthy fatty acids, such as those found in avocado, dried fruits, olive oil, and other vegetable-based oils, helps to strengthen the outer layer of cells, making it more difficult for viruses to enter.

Antioxidants are molecules that aid in the defense of the organism against harmful agents and the state of oxidative stress.

Which is the most crucial?

Glutathione is a substance produced by our bodies and found in a variety of foods such as avocado, spinach, peaches, and apples. Then there are foods that stimulate Glutathione production, such as garlic, onion, red fruits and vegetables, which are high in Selenium.

Vitamin C is found in high concentrations in all green vegetables, berries, and citrus fruits; because it has a higher bioavailability, it is best to get this vitamin from fresh foods rather than supplements.

Vitamin D deficiency is directly linked to an ineffective immune system; recent surveys have revealed that over 70% of the world's population is vitamin D deficient. It's abundant in vegetables, particularly mushrooms.

Carrots, pumpkin, parsley, ripe tomatoes, broccoli, and green cabbage are high in B-carotene (a precursor to Vitamin A) "..

Other micronutrients useful for keeping the immune system efficient and ready to react to external "aggressions" include selenium, zinc, and copper, which are found in legumes, mushrooms, and almonds and are important metals for their antioxidant activity.

Because they are high in fiber, probiotics and prebiotics found in all fruits and vegetables keep the microbiota healthy.

As you may have noticed, these are the same ingredients that make up the foundation of an alkaline and anti-inflammatory diet.

IT'S EASY TO INCLUDE A PLANT-BASED DIET IN YOUR LIFESTYLE.

How to properly balance your meals throughout the day

It's simple because a plant-based diet is diverse and abundant in foods that give the nutrients the body needs to operate optimally:

Fibers such as whole grains, which are preferable if naturally gluten-free, proteins mostly from legumes, healthy fats derived from dried fruit, vitamins and minerals from nature's numerous fruits and vegetables

In 2014, the Vegan Plate was published in the Journal of the Academy of Nutrition and Dietetics, a very helpful tool that helps you to correctly organize your plant nutrition in order to consume all of the nutrients essential to keep us healthy. With over 25000 members, this nutritionist organization is one of the biggest and most prominent in the world. Anyone may download the article for free.

The Vegan Plate is a fantastic visual depiction based only on plant meals that may maintain the proper balance of all the vital nutritional components that our bodies need. Fruits, vegetables, nuts, oilseeds, lipids, and proteins are the six primary dietary categories that include these vital components.

We placed nutritional ingredients high in vitamin B12 and vitamin D in the middle of the plate to underline the relevance of these two vitamins in a well balanced plant diet. It is crucial to begin by calculating one's daily calorie needs. These needs vary based on whether you are a man or a woman, the sort of employment you do, and the amount of physical activity you engage in.

Once the daily calorie needs have been calculated, the vegan plate may simply be split into the six food groups listed above.

So, instead of using scales or calorie computations to figure out what to put on your plate, just follow the vegan plate's easy and helpful guidelines.

To properly distribute meals throughout the day, they should be divided into three major meals with one or two snacks in between.

Breakfast like a king, lunch like a middle-class person, and supper like a poor, according to an ancient adage.

Breakfast should consist of a decent herbal tea, vegetable milk, or coffee. If you like, you may add bitter cocoa or dark chocolate crumbles to a porridge made with whole cereal flakes, vegetarian yogurt, dried fruit, and chia seeds. A fruit may be eaten to round out your morning.

Fruit, such as berries with low fructose content, or dried fruit, slices of dry coconut, or high-quality dark chocolate chips, should be included in snacks.

Lunch and supper should contain a substantial number of vegetables, ideally fresh but also cooked or merely blanched, in order to provide the necessary nutrients. You will be able to receive all of the required enzymes to better tackle digestion if you start your meal with vegetables; also, since vegetables have a satiating capacity, you will be more likely to finish the meal without caloric excesses. Lunch may also be followed with a meal made with gluten-free cereals, particularly whole wheat, or a dish made with vegetable proteins such those found in legumes.

The following is a list of gluten-free cereals or gluten-free cereals that include a particularly digestible kind of gluten, such as spelt:

Amaranth

rice that is black in color

Kamut

Quinoa

Rya

Emmer

Rice that has been harvested from the wild

During the day, herbal teas brewed with the plants listed below are recommended:

Raspberry red Alvaca Clove Chamomille Anice Fennel Ginger

Tea made with sea moss

Lemongrass

Using spices as an ingredient in all of one's foods is also highly advised. The following is a list of healthful spices with descriptions of their properties:

Curcumin is an antioxidant that benefits brain, cardiovascular, and joint health. Dandelion is a blood and liver purifier.

Elderberry (Sambucus nigra) - helps to protect the body against colds. Burdock root is a blood and liver cleanser that also acts as a diuretic.

Vitamin and mineral supplements made from bladderwrack (seaweed). Bromelain and papain are enzymes that break down proteins in the small intestine.

Proteins, vitamins and minerals, and detoxifiers are all found in chlorella (seaweed). Vitamin and mineral supplements made from Irish moss (seaweed).

Antiviral oregano oil

Blood cleanser, antibacterial, anti-inflammatory, and diuretic sarsaparilla Parasite-killing wormwood leaf

Vitamin and mineral supplements made from kelp (seaweed).

Flaxseed - rich essential fatty acids, prevents heart disease, cancer, and diabetes

Breakfast ideas that are both healthy and delicious

Cappuccino with soy milk

Two pieces of whole wheat spelt bread with a spread of creamy dried fruit like hazelnuts, almonds, or pistachios, as well as thin slices of fresh fruit like bananas

a cup of espresso

A cup of white vegetable yogurt topped with cereal flakes, chopped almonds, and sliced fresh fruit. Flax or chia seeds, which are high in omega 3 fatty acids, may be sprinkled on top.

Lunch as an example

Pitas with chickpea hummus, olives, and green leafy veggies on top. These veggies are exceptionally high in calcium, allowing individuals who follow a plant-based diet to meet their calcium needs without ingesting dairy products.

Apple slices with cinnamon and almond cream on top.

Dinner as an example

Quinoa with cooked peas and finely sliced zucchini

Avocado and walnut salad with flax seed oil dressing.

Sport and a plant-based diet

Sporting exercise is beneficial for more than simply weight loss and body sculpting. It's first and foremost a health-related decision.

To perform effective sports activity, we must understand how to feed our bodies with "clean" meals that give us with the required energy and aid in the recovery of our bodies after we have participated in sports.

Many well-known athletes, such as Carl Lewis, have shown that a plant-based diet may help them attain high levels of athletic performance.

Those who consume a vegetable-based diet do well in sports and, more importantly, recover rapidly after engaging in physical exercise.

The lactic acid produced by the body adds to the feeling of exhaustion experienced while participating in sports.

Because the tissues are already alkaline, the body creates less lactic acid while eating a plant-based diet, and the lactic acid created by the body under stress is "buffered" and disposed of more rapidly.

Plant foods having a high protein content, such as beans, are recommended for athletes. The legumes with the greatest protein are:

soybeans

beans in a wide sense

lupins

Even among cereals, those with a greater protein content are preferable:

oats

amaranth\sspelt

quinoa\sbuckwheat

Finally, oilseeds and dried fruits have a high protein content: There are a few that are particularly high in protein: linseeds, pumpkin seeds

seeds of sesame

pinecones

almonds

Spirulina, which is high in protein and iron, is the most well-known "doping" for athletes who consume veggies.

So, there are a few secrets to improving athletic performance: all you have to do is know them!

HOW TO EMPOWER YOURSELF WITH A PLANT-BASED DIET

Step one: INCLUDE THOSE FOODS IN YOUR DAILY DIET THAT HAVE BEEN CLASSIFIED AS SUPERFOODS BY THE MEDICAL-SCIENTIFIC LITERATURE.

Avocado is a powerhouse of beneficial nutrients. It's high in potassium and magnesium, mineral salts that play a role in all cellular interactions; it's also high in fiber and fatty acids. Our bodies can simply employ the latter to make energy, avoiding insulin surges that contribute to body fat buildup. Avocado has been found in recent research to be effective in preventing cancer, particularly stomach and pancreatic cancer, combating osteoporosis, and reducing the symptoms of depression.

Blueberries and red fruits are high in antioxidants, which reduce cellular aging. They also have a purifying and anti-inflammatory activity, which helps decrease blood sugar levels, and they encourage the rise of good HDL cholesterol, which strengthens the whole cardiovascular system. Despite their low sugar content, they are a concentrated source of taste that should not be overlooked in smoothies or salads....

Cumin: A spice with a strong scent that originates from the seeds of a herbaceous plant; high in calcium, magnesium, phosphorus, vitamin A, and vitamin E; good for boosting the immune system and keeping harmful viruses at bay.

Cinnamon: Known for its aphrodisiac effect and ability to enhance flavors in the kitchen for more than 2000 years; rich in phenols that slow down the putrefaction of certain foods; regulates cholesterol levels, facilitates digestion, reduces blood glucose levels, enhances energy, and even has mood-boosting properties.

Cabbage and broccoli: Crucifers are cold-tolerant and high in antioxidants like vitamin K, vitamin A, vitamin E, magnesium, omega 3 fibers, iron, and potassium; a 100-gram serving of broccoli contains 150 percent of our daily vitamin C requirement; medical literature recognizes these plants as having strong anti-carcinogenic properties; they prevent diseases like diabetes and osteoporosis, fortify the immune system, and promote weaning. Raw or pan-seared is preferable.

Coconut oil is derived from the coconut fruit. Rich in MCT medium-chain triglycerides, which are more easily used by our bodies to produce energy than fats from animals, which are defined as long-chain; as a result, when you eat coconut, its fat is immediately oxidized by the liver, providing energy; as a result, it is very suitable for those who practice sports; however, it is also suitable for those who want to lose weight because, on the one hand, it prevents body fat accumulation and, on the other hand, it

Because of the lauric acid in it, it has significant antibacterial, viral, and fungal properties.

Turmeric is an antioxidant spice with potent anti-oxidant and anti-cancer properties, and it is widely used in holistic and ayurvedic medicine. Curcumin, the key component, has anti-inflammatory properties and is used to treat arthritis, inflammation, arthrosis, and joint discomfort. Turmeric also has the ability to protect the immune system.

Chocolate: It must include a high proportion of cocoa, at least 80%, and be raw if possible. It is recommended that you eat no more than 30 grams of sugar every day.

The term "food of gods" is used to describe chocolate. It's abundant in:

Antioxidants in magnesium

Tryptophan is a vital amino acid that helps to calm the nervous system and enhance the quality of sleep. It also contains polyphenols, which help to boost brain function and decrease cognitive decline. Blood pressure and cholesterol are controlled by flavonoids, which preserve the interior wall of blood vessels.

You'll discover some delicious chocolate-based desserts in the recipes section!

Step two:

Chapter 3

ADD DIETARY SUPPLEMENTS ON A DAILY BASIS OR IN CYCLES

It may be useful to augment the plaint based diet with various dietary supplements to enhance the favorable benefits.

Vitamin B-12 (cobalamin)

Vitamin B-12 is required for the proper functioning of blood and brain cells, as well as the creation of DNA.

People who eat a vegan or vegetarian diet, as well as those who are older, are at risk of acquiring B-12 deficiency.

Fatigue, depression, tingling in the hands and feet, and anemia are all symptoms of B-12 insufficiency.

Essential Fatty Acids Omega-3

Omega-3 essential fatty acids are essentially made up of the different components of cell membranes. They are beneficial in the following areas:

ADD DIETARY SUPPLEMENTS ON A DAILY BASIS OR IN CYCLES

sustaining healthy heart health and a good cardio circulatory system brain functioning and visual health energy

Vitamin C, often known as ascorbic acid, is a water-soluble vitamin.

Although a plant-based diet is abundant in vitamin-rich foods, it is still necessary to include this vitamin since today's agricultural soils are less fertile than those of the past, and as a result, fruits may not contain as much vitamin C as they formerly did.

We're also talking about a vitamin that is rapidly degraded by heat, so we aren't always able to absorb it in the proper amounts.

Because it is involved in so many metabolic and enzymatic activities, it is one of the most essential vitamins:

Strengthens immunological defenses, improving immune cells' capacity to create antibodies and hence the body's ability to better withstand all illnesses.

It aids in the detoxification of the body (toxins resulting from smoke or pollution).

By altering collagen formation, it protects and restores tissues; the latter protects the functions of cartilage, bones, skin, capillaries, and gums.

It is an antioxidant because it counteracts the detrimental effects of free radicals, or chemicals that promote premature aging in our bodies.

It is beneficial in the event of anemia because it enhances iron digestion, which is a crucial mineral for the synthesis of red blood cells.

It reduces stress by assisting in the creation of chemicals that maintain nerve impulse transmission steady, as well as regulating the manufacture of the stress hormone.

Vitamin D is an important nutrient.

Our bodies can only create vitamin D when they are exposed to sunlight.

It may be beneficial to include this vitamin in one's diet if they are infrequently exposed to the sun or just during specific seasons of the year.

This vitamin is vital for the following reasons:

Because it aids in maintaining an appropriate level of calico in the blood, it is necessary for proper mineralization of bones and teeth.

To support the health of our kidneys, arteries, and bodily tissues; to improve the immune system against illnesses and viruses

ADD DIETARY SUPPLEMENTS ON A DAILY BASIS OR IN CYCLES

Maintaining the heart's and cardio-circulatory system's functioning.

Step three: CHOOSE HIGH-QUALITY FOOD AND AVOID GENETICALLY MODIFIED FOOD.

Because this is a detox diet, it's preferable to choose organic or sustainable bio food that's free of chemicals and heavy metals to maximum efficacy.

Step four is to:

DRINK A LOT OF WATER, PREFERABLY SPRING WATER.

Drinking lots of water every day is crucial since water is necessary for a healthy and efficient body; also, water aids in nutrient absorption.

Drinking spring water would be excellent.

Water that runs from rocks or deep soils is known as spring water, and it is a dynamic, active, and vital element.

As a result, spring water has a rich and pleasant flavor. It hydrates and refreshes us better than tap water or other forms of water.

If the source is alpine, the water is filtered by earthy and sandy layers that work as a filter, preventing heavy contaminants from entering the water; as a result, we are dealing with waters that are normally quite pure.

It's also referred to as 'dynamized water,' which is water that has the power to energize the body's cells while also being beneficial to the excretory organs like the kidneys and liver.

When purchasing spring water, ensure sure the source's name and location, as well as a statement of bottling at the source, are put on the bottle label.

FOOD: THE ORIGINAL ANTI-DISEASE MEDICINE

Weight loss with a plant-based diet

We've seen how a plant-based diet may improve health by preventing and curing major illnesses.

Is it, however, causing you to lose weight?

When it comes to losing weight, even this sort of diet must adhere to the concept of calorie deficit: no deficit, no weight loss. While it isn't a diet's credo, it is the "hidden" idea at the heart of all weight-loss diets.

Weight reduction is a natural result of following a plant-based diet since the foods it comprises are often low in calories and satiating due to their high water and dietary fiber content.

The accumulation of body fat, particularly in the belly, is a precursor to the onset of various illnesses such as diabetes, autoimmune disorders, and oncological diseases.

ADD DIETARY SUPPLEMENTS ON A DAILY BASIS OR IN CYCLES

As a result, it's critical not to dismiss this early signal from the body and to act quickly to get the metabolic system back on track.

To this purpose, a plant-based diet is beneficial since it has many fibers that have a satiating and fulfilling impact, allowing us to go longer without feeling hungry; it also contains little saturated fats.

Neurodegenerative illness and a plant-based diet

Food is made up of chemical and biological molecules that interact with our cells, including neurons, and may have a positive or negative influence depending on the quality of the food we consume.

Neurons are unable to replicate and regenerate if all cells reproduce and renew. They have the ability to rejuvenate but not reproduce. As a result, it is preferable to safeguard them as much as possible, particularly after they reach a certain age.

Mercury, lead, and other environmentally hazardous ions accumulate specifically in adipose tissue and nerve tissue with a fat component.

Chronic inflammation may contribute to the beginning and progression of neurodegenerative disorders like Alzheimer's and dementia, which are becoming more common: the central nervous system is composed up of neurons that, when inflamed, cause the nervous system to malfunction.

The good news is that nature always provides us with solutions. We may opt to consume "The Magnificent Seven," a group of entirely vegetarian meals that nourish and maintain the central nervous system.

Let's practice using them all on a daily basis:

Green tea tastes better when had first thing in the morning.

When ginger and turmeric are used as fresh roots, they are more effective.

Dark chocolate tastes better when it is processed raw, which implies that the cocoa beans used to make chocolate must not have been heated over 42 degrees.

Berries are high in vitamins, minerals, and polyphenols and provide a lot of them.

Dried fruits, with the exception of peanuts, which are allergenic and inflammatory. Walnuts are chosen because their form resembles that of our brain. They are anti-inflammatory and high in omega 3.

Flax seeds, chia seeds, and hemp seeds are all good sources of omega-3 fatty acids.

Chlorella tea is a freshwater alga that has powerful cleansing properties.

Conclusion

ADD DIETARY SUPPLEMENTS ON A DAILY BASIS OR IN CYCLES

Maintaining a diet over time and keeping it sustainable seems to be far more difficult than getting started on one. While most individuals stick to a diet for a short amount of time, until they achieve their objectives, converting the diet into a new eating regimen to include into their lifestyle is exceedingly challenging.

A tactic called as "crowding out" is one approach to persuade us to eat healthier meals. It's simple: instead of removing unhealthy items from your diet, you can just incorporate better ones. Consider the following scenario:

You can gradually incorporate new healthy eating habits: the more often you eat healthy meals, the more likely you are to become accustomed to them and eventually prefer them to harmful ones; you can start the meal with a certain amount of raw vegetables: this will increase satiety and alkalize the meal; you can gradually incorporate new healthy eating habits: the more often you eat healthy meals, the more likely you are to become accustomed to them and eventually start preferring them to harmful ones. It only takes a few weeks to form a new habit; it is preferable to go shopping when you are not hungry: When we buy food when we aren't hungry, we make impulsive choices that aren't particularly reasonable; keep in mind that choosing veggie food is an ethical and environmentally sustainable decision.

If our health is excellent or if we already have diseases, switching to a plant-based diet can only bring one thing if we place ourselves in the best possible situation: the ability to heal ourselves. benefits. It's important to realize that our bodies are quite powerful.

Numerous scientific studies have shown that a healthy diet may prevent various ailments and, in many instances, cure them till they go away completely.

However, many individuals are unwilling to prioritize a healthy lifestyle in their everyday lives. People who suffer from chronic diseases are often those who consume foods that inflame their bodies on a regular basis, don't commit enough time to exercise, and live in constant tension, unable to cleanse their bad thoughts with a few minutes of meditation or deep relaxation each day.

In a future book, I'd want to go through all of these issues in more depth.

For the time being, I was content to share what I had learned about clean, green, anti-inflammatory, and healing diet with you.

I genuinely hope I was able to demonstrate how much we can improve the quality of our lives by just "consuming" what we have selected with conscience and knowledge, rather than what is easily accessible.

ADD DIETARY SUPPLEMENTS ON A DAILY BASIS OR IN CYCLES

Continued success on your own path toward a more "conscious" diet!

RECIPES The following recipes are a collection of simple to make meals that show that healthy eating can be delicious as well.

And now, good luck with your meal!

Lasagna with carasau bread – cover picture – Preparation time: 20 minutes

Time to prepare: 20 minutes

4 servings

Ingredients:

200 g pita bread or carasau bread Soy milk (700 mL)

almond flour (40 g) spinach, 400 g

spelt flour (70 g) Nutmeg, salt, and pepper

olive oil (extra virgin)

Preparation:

Boil the spinach, then remove it from the water and set it aside to cool.

In a separate saucepan, whisk together the flour and soy milk until well combined.

Season to taste with salt, pepper, and nutmeg.

Bring the béchamel sauce to a low boil, stirring constantly, until it becomes creamy. Allow time for cooling.

Add the spinach and two tablespoons of oil.

Form the layers of lasagna in a casserole dish by alternating the spinach cream with carasau bread that has been gently wet with a little water or soy milk. Add the almond flour in between each layer.

Serve with a piece of corasau bread on the side. Place in a preheated oven at 200 degrees for 20 minutes after adding a little oil.

Nutrition

350 calories per serving fat (4 g)

Carbohydrates: 59 g Protein: 19 g

Tartare with avocado, tofu, and asparagus

The preparation time is 20 minutes.

Time to cook: 10 minutes

2 servings

Ingredients:

250 grams of asparagus

Tofu, sliced into cubes, 80 g a single lime

4 tbsp olive oil (extra virgin) 40 pine nuts, lightly roasted

ADD DIETARY SUPPLEMENTS ON A DAILY BASIS OR IN CYCLES

a pinch of mustard powder seasoning with salt and pepper

garlic powder, a sprinkle basil leaves

Preparation:

Cook for 10 minutes with the asparagus.

Oil, garlic, half a lime juice, basil, and mustard powder should all be emulsified together.

To keep the avocado from darkening, dice it and sprinkle the remaining lime juice over it.

In a large mixing bowl, toss the chopped asparagus, avocado, and tofu with the oil emulsion.

Pour half of the compost into a ramekin that has been put in the middle of the dish to make the tartare.

Toasted pine nuts may be used as a garnish.

Nutrition

A serving has 440 calories and 35 grams of fat. Carbohydrates: 5,9 g Protein: 18 g

Crackers made with flaxseed

The preparation time is 20 minutes. Time to cook: 10 minutes

6 servings Ingredients:

200 g flour (millet or spelt) a teaspoon of dried chives 35 g extra virgin olive oil

Flax seeds, 60 g a teaspoon of salt and 200 mL of water

Preparation:

In a large mixing basin, combine all of the ingredients and mix with your hands until you have a homogenous dough.

Form the dough into a ball, cover it in plastic wrap, and place it in the refrigerator for two hours.

Preheat the oven to 200 degrees Fahrenheit.

On baking paper, roll out the dough into a rectangle with a relatively thin thickness.

Place the dough on an oven dish and cut it into cracker-sized pieces using a knife.

Preheat the oven to 350°F and bake for 10 minutes.

Remove the crackers from the oven and set them aside to cool before separating them.

Nutrition

195 calories per serving Fat content: 11 g Carbohydrates: 20 g Protein: 11 g

Casserole of Cabbage Rolls with a Twist

The preparation time is 10 minutes.

Time to cook: 40 minutes

4 servings

ADD DIETARY SUPPLEMENTS ON A DAILY BASIS OR IN CYCLES

Ingredients:

1 cup quinoa (cooked) a red onion and a half

2 garlic cloves, finely chopped four white mushrooms, minced

one and a half cans diced tomatoes, finely chopped 8 green cabbage leaves, whole teaspoons of extra virgin olive oil, vegetable stock or homemade vegetable broth cup of fresh basil leaves, minced

Instructions:

Preheat the oven to 350 degrees Fahrenheit (180 degrees Celsius).

In a non-stick pan, combine the extra virgin olive oil, onion, quinoa, garlic clove, and sliced mushrooms. 5 minutes in the oven Combine the tomato sauce, vegetable stock, and basil in a mixing bowl. Mix thoroughly. Cook for a further ten minutes.

2 cabbage leaves should be placed on top of the baking sheet. Place a quarter of the filling on top of the cabbage leaves and tie them together with kitchen twine. Make the next three rolls in the same manner.

Cover with aluminum foil and bake in the oven for 40 minutes.

Before serving, allow for a 10-minute resting time.

Nutrition

261 calories per serving fat (2 g)

Carbohydrates: 51 g Protein: 12 g

Mango, Quinoa, and Black Bean Casserole with a Tangy Sauce

The preparation time is 10 minutes.

Time to prepare: 25 minutes

4 servings

Ingredients:

coconut milk (two cups)

2 cups cooked quinoa 1 cup vegetable stock or homemade vegetable broth

Rinse and drain 2 cups black beans, rinsed and ready to use 1/4 cup fresh mint (minced) mango, peeled and chopped 1 peeled and chopped avocado

a pinch of pink Himalayan salt

extra virgin olive oil (teaspoons)

Instructions:

Preheat the oven to 425 degrees Fahrenheit (200 degrees Celsius).

In a casserole dish, combine the stock, milk, and quinoa and stir thoroughly.

Cover with aluminum foil and bake for 25 minutes.

ADD DIETARY SUPPLEMENTS ON A DAILY BASIS OR IN CYCLES

Remove the baking dish from the oven and turn it off. In a large mixing bowl, combine the beans, mango, avocado, and fresh mint.

Season with salt and olive oil before serving.

Nutrition

A serving has 573 calories. fat (23 g) Carbohydrates: 75 g protein (15 g)

Chapter 4

Onions with peppers Masala

The preparation time is 10 minutes.

Preparation time: 30 minutes

2 servings

Ingredients:

1 cup brown rice, uncooked 2 tblsp. coconut oil 1 tbsp cumin seeds, ground

1/2 teaspoon turmeric powder (freshly powdered) 2 peeled and finely chopped onions 2 nicely diced green chilies (1-inch) 1 slice of ginger, fresh

2 garlic cloves, grated

2 tbsp olive oil (extra virgin) 3 tblsp. tomato paste

1 tblsp. cayenne pepper

Himalayan pink salt, a pinch sliced and washed 1 red bell pepper, chopped

Instructions:

Cook for 25 to 30 minutes, or until the brown rice is done, in a small saucepan with enough boiling water to cover it over medium-low heat.

Meanwhile, in a nonstick pan, heat the coconut oil. Cumin seeds, turmeric, onion, garlic, chile, and ginger should all be added at this point. 5 minutes in the oven

Add the tomato paste and chili powder, as well as the salt. Mix everything well.

After you've added the bell pepper, cook for another 5 minutes.

Serve the rice immediately after tossing it with the hot masala.

Extra virgin olive oil is used to dress the salad.

Nutrition

520 calories per serving Carbohydrates: 81 milligrams

6 g dietary fiber 8 g fat

sugar (4 g) Protein: 4 g

Pizza with olives and basil

The preparation time is 10 minutes. Preparation time: 30 minutes Ingredients: Ingredients: Ingredients: Ingredients: Ingredients: Ingredients: Ingredients:

Use the following ingredients to make the pizza sauce:

1 can (15 oz.) chopped tomatoes 1 tbsp extra-virgin extra-virgin olive oil

2 garlic cloves, peeled and sliced 1/2 cup fresh basil leaves, properly washed

1 teaspoon powdered onion a quarter teaspoon of dried sage

1/4 teaspoon red chili flakes (optional) 1 teaspoon Himalayan pink salt

Use the following ingredients to make the pizza:

pita bread produced using flours that are allowed Vegan mozzarella, shredded (4 ounces).

Rinse and slice thinly 1 cup of your favorite mixed veggies (tomatoes; eggplant; onion; green pepper; mushroom)

1/3 cup pitted and finely chopped olives 1 tbsp extra-virgin extra-virgin olive oil

basil leaves, cleaned and broken up into little bits

Instructions:

Follow these instructions to make the sauce:

Mix on low until the basil and garlic are very little pieces in a blender, then add the olive oil and blend until smooth.

In a saucepan, combine the chopped tomatoes, onion powder, and salt and simmer for approximately 20 minutes, or until the sauce has reduced and thickened.

Follow these instructions to make the pizza:

Preheat the oven to 500 degrees F. Preheat oven to 350°F. Line a baking sheet with parchment paper and put aside.

Make a homogeneous coating of pizza sauce on the pitas. Sprinkle the sliced veggies and olives, the basil and garlic emulsion, and the dried sage on top of the vegan mozzarella.

Preheat oven to 350°F and bake for 8 minutes.

To finish, drizzle the pizzas with olive oil and scatter the basil leaves on top. Leftovers may be stored in an airtight container in the freezer for up to three weeks.

Nutrition

400 calories per serving Total fat: 10 g Carbohydrates: 64 milligrams

dietary fiber: 5 g sugar (2 g)

Protein: 10 g

Chili with black beans

Preparation time: 15 minutes Time to prepare: 20 minutes 2 servings

Ingredients:

coconut oil, 1 tablespoon

1 medium peeled and chopped onion 6 mushroom slices, cleaned and sliced

2 tblsp. coriander, freshly ground paprika (2 tablespoons)

cumin seeds, 2 tbsp.

1 tablespoon nutmeg, freshly grated 1 tblsp. red pepper flakes

1 can (15 oz.) chopped tomatoes 1 can black beans, rinsed

1 can kidney beans, washed

5 drained and washed cherry tomatoes 2 teaspoons pureed tomatoes

7 oz. brown rice, uncooked (optional)

4 tablespoons coconut yoghurt, to be used as a garnish (optional) 4 sprigs fresh cilantro, to be used as a garnish (optional)

Instructions:

In a large pan, melt the coconut oil over medium heat. Simmer for two minutes after adding the onion, then add the mushrooms and cook for another four minutes. Combine the coriander, paprika, cumin, cinnamon, and chili powder in a mixing bowl and mix thoroughly.

In a large mixing bowl, add the canned tomatoes and liquids, black beans, kidney beans, cherry tomatoes, and tomato purée. All of the ingredients should be combined and brought to a low simmer. Cook on medium heat for 25 minutes.

Prepare the rice according to the package instructions while the chilli cooks. After rinsing, drain.

Serve immediately with the chilli on top of the rice, topped with yoghurt (if using) and cilantro (if using).

Nutrition

Serving size: calorie count: calorie count: calorie count: calorie count: calorie count: Total fat: 580 5 g Carbohydrates: Dietary fiber (102 g) 14 g sugar, 14 g protein

Lentils come in a rainbow of hues.

15 minutes are necessary for preparation. Preparation time: 30 minutes 4 servings

Ingredients:

2 tblsp. coconut oil 1 peeled onion

2 peeled and coarsely chopped carrots 2 washed and sliced celery stalks

1 cleaned and sliced sweet potato 1 cup lentils, cooked

5 c. vegetable broth

Add a pinch of Himalayan pink salt to taste.

Instructions:

Heat the coconut oil over medium heat until it shimmers. Cook for 3 minutes after adding the onion.

Cook for another 2 minutes after adding the carrots, celery, and sweet potato to the other ingredients.

Combine the lentils and vegetable stock in a large mixing bowl. Stir regularly for approximately 25 minutes, or until the lentils are cooked.

Before serving, season with salt to taste.

Nutrition

330 calories per serving Carbohydrates: 49 g

10 g fat

fiber (20 g) Sugar content: 8 g

Protein content: 17 g

Pasta with Spelt and Tomatoes

15 minutes are necessary for preparation.

Time to prepare: 20 minutes

4 servings

ONIONS WITH PEPPERS MASALA

Ingredients:

Extra-virgin olive oil is a kind of extra-virgin olive oil that is (around 3 tablespoons) 2 peeled and crushed garlic cloves

1 onion, diced eggplant (rinsed and chopped) 2 peeled and sliced zucchinis or 3 cleaned and chopped tomatoes sun-dried tomatoes, 1 cup

2 tsp basil (dried) (optional)

1 tablespoon oregano leaves, dried 1 tbsp. balsamic vinegar

a pinch of pink Himalayan salt spelt spaghetti (7 ounces)

Instructions:

In a large pan over medium heat, shimmer the olive oil. 8 minutes, or until the eggplant is mushy, sauté the garlic, onion, and eggplant.

In a large mixing bowl, combine the zucchini, tomatoes, sun-dried tomatoes, basil, and oregano. Cook, stirring periodically, for 8 minutes. Season with salt and pepper.

Cook for about 10 minutes, or until the pasta is soft but not falling apart, in a separate pot with enough boiling water to cover it.

Serve the spaghetti with the sauce right away.

Nutrition

460 calories per serving Total fat: 12 g 75 g carbohydrate, 17 g protein 1 gram sugar

On a Stick: Crispy Green Tomatoes

The preparation time is 14 minutes.

Time to cook: 16 minutes

2 servings

Ingredients:

coconut flour, 1/4 cup 1 teaspoon of salt

4 green tomatoes, cut

1 cup applesauce (homemade) almond flour (1/2 cup)

extra-virgin olive oil, 1/4 cup

Instructions:

In a large mixing bowl, add the coconut flour and salt. Toss the tomatoes together in a large mixing bowl. Toss until all of the ingredients are evenly coated.

In a separate mixing bowl, pour the apple sauce. Add the almond flour and mix well. Mix everything together until it's completely smooth.

Toss in the oil and bring to a boil. Toss the tomatoes in the apple sauce combination and set aside. Carry on with the remaining tomatoes in the same manner. Fry the tomatoes in batches for approximately 3 minutes each, or until golden brown. Serve.

Nutrition

Serving size: calorie count: calorie count: calorie count: calorie count: calorie count: 113 4.2 g fat

0.8 g saturated fat 0 milligrams of cholesterol

861 milligrams sodium

22.5 g carbohydrate

6.3 g fiber

2.3 g sugar

9.2 g protein

Cider-based fruit salad

The preparation time is 11 minutes.

Time to cook: 16 minutes

3 servings

Ingredients:

diced apple, little Grapefruit pulp, chopped into bite-sized bits 1 small apricot, cubed teaspoons apple cider vinegar, warmed in the microwave 1/4 cup jacamar, cubed 1 tablespoon of apple cider vinegar sauce a sprinkle of cinnamon powder, ground

Instructions:

In a small mixing bowl, combine the apple cider vinegar and cinnamon powder.

In a large mixing bowl, combine the salad ingredients with the cider sauce, apple cider vinegar, and cinnamon. Toss everything together thoroughly, then divide the mixture evenly among the plates. As quickly as feasible, serve.

Nutrition

Each serving has 123 calories. 14.2 g of fat

0.7 g saturated fat 14.2 g total fat 0 milligrams of cholesterol

661 milligrams sodium

22.5 g carbohydrate, 6.3 g dietary fiber Sugar content: 0 g

Protein content: 9.2 g

Zucchini and Broccoli Stir-Fry

15 minutes are necessary for preparation.

Time to prepare: 15 minutes

4 servings

Ingredients:

ONIONS WITH PEPPERS MASALA

2 teaspoons each of coconut oil and sesame oil, peeled and coarsely chopped fresh ginger 4 peeled garlic cloves, minced onions (rinsed and chopped)

1 broccoli head, cleaned and florets separated

3-scallions, peeled and coarsely chopped 1-cup steaming zucchini, cleaned and split into long strips

1 tablespoon basil leaves, finely chopped coconut amino acid, 1 oz

Instructions:

In a wok or large pan, heat the coconut and sesame oils over medium heat. Combine the ginger and garlic in a bowl. 5 minutes in the oven

In the same pan, add the onions and broccoli and cook for 3 minutes, or until the onion softens a little.

Combine the zucchini, scallions, and basil in a large mixing bowl. Toss all of the ingredients together and cook for 4 minutes, or until the vegetables are soft and delicious.

Remove from the heat, add the coconut amino, and place on a serving platter.

Nutrition

180 calories per serving Total fat: 14 g Carbohydrates: 13 grams

dietary fiber: 3 g sugar (4 g)

Protein: 3 g

Pesto-Smothered Kamut Noodles

5 minutes are required for preparation.

Time to prepare: 15 minutes

2 servings

Ingredients:

Extra-virgin olive oil is a kind of extra-virgin olive oil that is (around 3 tablespoons) 1 bunch basil leaves, freshly picked

6 cups cooked kamut noodles, well washed (cooked according to package directions) 1 bunch parsley (fresh)

1 bunch cilantro (fresh)

a pinch of pink Himalayan salt

Instructions:

In a blender, combine the olive oil, basil, parsley, and cilantro until smooth. Blend until the mixture is smooth.

Combine the cooked noodles and the sauce in a large mixing basin. Toss to combine flavours.

Nutrition

Calories in a serving: 355 Total fat: 21

Carbohydrates: 36 g Dietary fiber: 1 g Protein: 9 g

Quinoa Bowl

The preparation time is 10 minutes. Time required for cooking: 10 minutes Ingredients: Ingredients: Ingredients: Ingredients: Ingredients: Ingredients: Ingredients:

1 cup of quinoa, well washed\scup of water brought to a boil 1 can black beans, rinsed One teaspoon of cumin seeds, 2 minced garlic cloves,\slimes (squeezed) (squeezed) Avocado thinly sliced

Fresh cilantro (about one handful) (about one handful)

Instructions:

Pour the quinoa inside the boiling water and mix. Cook it for about 8 minutes.

While that's happening, in a small skillet combine the black beans, scallions, garlic, cumin and lime juice.

Simmer for 10 minutes.

Combine the quinoa and warmed beans in a large mixing basin until well combined. Place the avocado and cilantro over the top and serve immediately.

Nutrition

420 calories per serving 9 g of total fat Carbohydrates: 70 g\s18 g of dietary fibre sugar (2 g)

Protein: 10 g

Roasted vegetables

The preparation time is 14 minutes.

Cooking time: 17 minutes

2 servings

Ingredients:

2 cups of olive oil, 2 heads of big garlic 2 big eggplants

2 large shallots peeled, then quartered 2 carrots, peeled and cut into cubes

1 giant parsnip, peeled and cut into cubes 1 small green bell pepper

1 broccoli

1 big sprig of thyme, with leaves plucked A pinch of salt

Ingredients for garnishing

½ lemon divided into wedges and ½ squeezed 1 / 8 cup fennel bulb, finely chopped

Instructions:

Preheat the oven until the temperature reaches 425 degrees Fahrenheit.

Prepare a deep roasting pan by lining it with aluminum foil and gently greasing it with oil. Toss in all the vegetables, herbs and salt to taste.

Add the remaining oil and lemon juice until well combined. Toss everything together well.

To cover the roasting pan, place a piece of aluminum foil. Place this on the center oven rack and bake for 30 minutes. Remove the aluminum foil from the pan. After cooling for a few minutes, divide evenly among plates.

Finish with a fennel bulb, finely chopped and a slice of lemon for garnish. Before you begin to eat, squeeze the lemon juice over the top of the meal.

Nutrition

Calories in a serving: 164 4.2 g fat

0.8 g saturated fat

Cholesterol: 0 milligrams

Sodium: 861 milligrams

22.5 g carbohydrate, 6.3 g dietary fiber Sugar: 23 g

9.2 grams of protein

Pilaf Emmer

The preparation time is 10 minutes.

Time to prepare: 15 minutes

4 servings

Ingredients:

1 cup of emmer filtered water

4 cleaned, seeded, and chopped tomatoes Extra-virgin olive oil is a kind of extra-virgin olive oil that is (around 2 tablespoons) 1/4 cup of chopped dried apricot\s1 teaspoon grated lemon zest 1 tbsp. lemon juice

1/2 cup of finely chopped fresh parsley (rinsed and chopped) (rinsed and chopped) a pinch of pink Himalayan salt

Instructions:

Place the emmer and tomatoes in a pot full of water. Boil for 15 minutes and drain.

Combine the olive oil, apricots, lemon zest, lemon juice, and parsley in a large mixing bowl. Adjust seasonings if needed, and serve.

Nutrition

Serving size: calorie count: calorie count: calorie count: calorie count: calorie count: 270 Fat: 8 g

Carbohydrates: 42 g dietary fiber: 5 g 3 g of sugar

6 g of protein

ONIONS WITH PEPPERS MASALA

Chapter 5

Onions with a sweet and sour taste

The preparation time is 10 minutes.

Cooking time: 11 minutes

4 servings

Ingredients:

A vegetable stock or homemade vegetable broth 6 big onions halved\s2 garlic cloves crushed

1/2 tablespoon of balsamic vinegar 1/2 teaspoon of Dijon mustard

1 tablespoon agave syrup

Instructions:

In a large skillet, combine the onions and garlic. Fry for 3 minutes or until the vegetables are tender.

Combine the stock, vinegar, Dijon mustard, and agave syrup.

Make sure the heat is turned down. Simmer the mixture under a cover for 10 minutes.

Remove yourself from the heat. Continue stirring after the liquid has been reduced and the onions have become brown. Serve.

Nutrition

203 calories per serving Fat: 41.2 g

Saturated Fat: 0.8 g Sodium: 861 milligrams

Carbohydrates: 29.5 g\s16.3 g of dietary fiber

29.3 g of sugar

19.2 grams of protein

Apples and Onions Sautéed with Olive Oil

The preparation time is 14 minutes.

Time to cook: 16 minutes

2 servings

Ingredients:

2 cups of unsweetened apple cider 1 big onion, peeled and halved

A vegetable stock

4 apples, peeled and cut into wedges A pinch of sea salt

Instructions:

In a medium-sized pot, combine the cider and onion. Cook until the onions are soft and the liquid has dried.

Put in the stock and apples, seasoning with salt to taste Cook them for approximately 10 minutes. Serve.

Nutrition

Calories in a serving : 343 Total fat: 50.12 g 0.8 g saturated fat Cholesterol: 0 milligrams

Sodium: 861 milligrams

22.5 g carbohydrate

6.3 g of dietary fiber

2.3 g of sugar

9.2 g of protein

Zucchini Noodles with Portobello Mushrooms

The preparation time is 14 minutes.

Time to cook: 16 minutes

2 servings

Ingredients:

ONIONS WITH A SWEET AND SOUR TASTE

zucchini, shredded and made into spaghetti-like strands 3 garlic cloves, peeled and minced\sfinely sliced white onions (optional) (optional) 1 inch of julienned ginger

2 pounds of portobello mushrooms, cut into thick slivers Pinch of sea salt

2 table spoons of sesame oil 2 tblsp. coconut oil

1/4 cup finely chopped fresh chives (for garnish) (for garnish)

Instructions:

Melt 2 tablespoons of coconut oil over medium heat in a saucepan. Cook mushroom slivers for 5 minutes or until brown.

Add the onion, garlic, and ginger and cook for three minutes, until the onion is soft.

Bring the water to a boil. Reduce the heat gradually and allow the zucchini to simmer for 1 minute, drain and add the onion and mushroom sauce and sesame oil.

To serve, divide the zucchini noodles into equal portions and arrange them in individual dishes. Top the dish with chives.

Nutrition

163 calories in a serving Saturated fat is present: 0.8 g Cholesterol: 0 milligrams

Sodium: 861 milligrams

22.5 g carbohydrate

6.3 g of dietary fiber Sugar content: 0 g

4.2 grams of protein

Tempeh with Pineapple on the Grill

Time required for preparation: 12 minutes

Time to cook: 16 minutes

2 servings

Ingredients:

1 package tempeh (10 ounces, sliced) (10 ounces, sliced) 1/4 pineapple, cut into rings

coconut oil, 1 tablespoon

Orange juice (about 2 tablespoons, freshly squeezed) (about 2 tablespoons, freshly squeezed), Freshly squeezed lemon juice (about 1 tablespoon),\s1 tablespoon of extra virgin olive oil

Instructions:

Combine the olive oil, orange and lemon juice and coconut oil in a large mixing bowl until well combined. Put the tempeh to marinate in the bowl for e few minutes.

Heat a grill pan over medium-high heat until hot. Lift the marinated tempeh out of the bowl with a pair of tongs and place it on the grill pan after it has reached a high temperature.

Grill for 2 to 3 minutes.

Slice the pineapples, grill it for a few minutes and place them on a serving plate.

Place the grilled tempeh and pineapple on a serving tray. As quickly as feasible, serve.

Nutrition

163 calories per serving Saturated fat is present: 0.8 g Cholesterol: 0 milligrams

Sodium: 861 milligrams

22.5 g carbohydrate

6.3 g of dietary fiber Sugar content: 0 g

9.2 grams of protein

Courgettes with Apple Cider Sauce

The preparation time is 10 minutes.

Cooking time: 17 minutes

2 servings

Ingredients:

2 cups of baby courgettes (cut in half) (cut in half) 3 tbsp. of vegetable stock (optional) (optional)

2 tbsp. of apple cider vinegar (optional) (optional) 1 tablespoon light brown sugar (optional) (optional) Onions, thinly cut (about 4) (about 4)

A piece of grated ginger root (fresh or dried) (fresh or dried) 1 tablespoon of quinoa flour

2 teaspoons of water

Instructions:

To begin grill the courgette slices

While that's going on, in a saucepan, add the vegetable stock, apple cider vinegar, brown sugar, onions, ginger root. Bring the mixture to a boil. Reduce the heat to low and allow for 3 minutes of simmering.

Combine the quinoa flour and water in a mixing bowl. Make a thorough stir. Pour the sauce into the saucepan.

Put the courgettes in a serving dish. Add the onion source and le quinoa cream over the top.

Nutrition

Calories: 173 per serving

9.2 g of total fat

Saturated fat is present: 0.8 g Cholesterol: 0 milligrams

Sodium: 861 milligrams

22.5 g carbohydrate

Fiber: 6.3\sSugar: 2.3 g

9.2 grams of protein

Baked Mixed Mushrooms

Time required for preparation: 8 minutes

Time to prepare: 20 minutes

2 servings

Ingredients:

2 cups of mixed mushrooms 2 shallots\sgarlic cloves

cups of toasted chopped pecans 2 sprigs of fresh thyme

bunch of flat-leaf parsley\stablespoons of extra-virgin olive oil 2 bay leaves

1/2 cup of stale spelled bread

Instructions:

Finely chop the garlic once it has been peeled.

Chop the mixed mushrooms into small pieces. Wash them well. Pick the thyme leaves and tear the bread into tiny pieces with your fingers.

Pick the parsley leaves and coarsely chop them in a bowl.

Cook it for 12 minutes shallots, mixed mushrooms, oil and garlic. Add thyme, bay leaves and adjust the flavor as needed. Cook another 5 minutes.

Transfer the mushroom mixture to a 20 cm by 25 cm baking dish that has been covered with aluminum foil.

Add pecans and parsley on the top.

Bake for 35 minutes at 350°F in the oven. After that, remove the foil and continue to cook for another 10 minutes. Serve the finished dish with toast spelled bread.

Nutrition

Calories in a serving: 343 Total fat: 4.3

0.8 g saturated fat Cholesterol: 0 milligrams

Sodium: 861 milligrams

22.5 g carbohydrate

6.3 g of fiber, Sugar: 2.3\s

9.2 grams of protein

With a Spicy Twist on Okra

The preparation time is 14 minutes.

Time to cook: 16 minutes

2 servings

ONIONS WITH A SWEET AND SOUR TASTE

Ingredients:

2 cups okra 1/2 teaspoon turmeric, freshly ground

2 tablespoons fresh coriander, freshly chopped 1 tablespoon ground cumin seeds

a quarter teaspoon of salt

1 tablespoon coconut desiccated

3 tbsp olive oil (extra virgin) 1/2 teaspoon mustard seeds, black a teaspoon of coconut oil and 1/2 teaspoon of cumin seeds

2 fresh tomatoes to top it off

Instructions:

Trim the okra to the length you want it. Rinse and dry completely.

Combine the turmeric, fresh coriander, cumin, salt, and desiccated coconut in a mixing bowl and stir well.

Cook the mustard and cumin seeds in a pan with coconut oil for 3 minutes to ensure they are aromatic. Toss in the okra. Combine the spices in a bowl. On a low heat setting, cook for 8 minutes.

Place the mixture on a platter to serve. If desired, garnish with sliced fresh tomatoes.

Nutrition

183 calories per serving, 4 g fats

Saturated fat: 0.8 g 0 milligrams of cholesterol

861 milligrams sodium 22.5 g carbohydrate

6.3 g fiber

2.3 g sugar

9.2 g protein

Green Soup with Alkalinizing Effects

The preparation time is 10 minutes.

Time to prepare: 10 minutes

2 servings

Ingredients:

1 tablespoon coconut oil 1 pint sweet potatoes in stock

fennel seeds, 1/4 teaspoon a red onion and a half

2 broccoli stems

4 cups spinach (baby) (drained)

1 tblsp lemon juice + zest

1 peeled and roughly chopped garlic clove

Instructions:

Over medium heat, saute the garlic, red onions, and fennel seeds in a little oil for about 2 minutes.

Simmer for 4 minutes, stirring regularly, with the broccoli, lemon zest, stock, and lemon juice.

Remove the skillet from the heat after the spinach has wilted.

Transfer the ingredients to a blender right away and mix until fully smooth and creamy.

Nutrition

218 calories per serving

Fat content: 7.2 g 3.8 g saturated fat

Cholesterol in the amount of 3 milligrams 801 milligrams sodium 12.5 g carbohydrates

3.3 g fiber

Soup with Carrots and Ginger

The preparation time is 10 minutes.

Time to prepare: 15 minutes

2 servings

Ingredients:

a tablespoon of freshly grated ginger 1/4 onion, 1/2 tablespoon salt, garlic cloves

4 peeled carrots, cut into pieces 2 liters of vegetable broth 1 tsp turmeric

Instructions:

Bring all of the ingredients to a boil and cook for an hour.

Allow it to cool.

Using an immersion blender, blend them together until they're smooth and creamy.

Sprinkle hemp seeds on top of the dish as a garnish if preferred.

Nutrition

210 calories per serving

Fat content: 8.2 g Saturated fat: 3.8 g cholesterol milligrams 801 milligrams sodium 12.5 g carbohydrates

5.3 g fiber

Kale salad (salad de kale)

The preparation time is 10 minutes.

Time to cook: 5 minutes

2 servings

Ingredients:

1 medium avocado, sliced

cleaned, dried, and thinly cut kale head 1 tomato, medium

For the purpose of dressings

a couple of teaspoons extra-virgin olive oil 1 teaspoon mustard (Dijon) (optional) 4 drops stevia liquid extract

lemon juice, 1 tbsp.

Among the garnishes are:

a handful of pumpkin seeds

Tempeh that has been seared in a few pieces

Instructions:

Combine all of the dressing ingredients in a bowl and use to coat the kale.

Place the avocado and greens in a salad bowl.

Season with salt and pepper and serve with toppings.

Nutrition

248 calories per serving 4.2 g fat

2.8 g saturated fat

0.5 milligrams of cholesterol (mg) 813 milligrams sodium

13.5 g carbohydrates

3.3 g fiber

Turmeric Curry with Roasted Cauliflower

The preparation time is 10 minutes.

Time to prepare: 35 minutes

4 servings

Before we get started, it's important to note that this meal includes four of the most powerful anti-inflammatory ingredients available: bell pepper, turmeric, ginger, and garlic.

Coconut oil, seeds, and almonds contribute to the meal's healthful fat content. As a result, you may be certain that when you eat this meal, you are providing tremendous service to your body's immune system.

Ingredients:

powdered turmeric (about 1 teaspoon) 1 and 1/2 cups water 1 teaspoon Himalayan salt chili powder (1/2 teaspoon)

cauliflower florets, sliced into pieces

1 tablespoon finely chopped coriander Coconut milk, unsweetened (about 2 cups) 2 tblsp. coconut oil

1 peeled and chopped garlic clove 1 teaspoon powdered ginger

almonds, 1/2 cup

Instructions:

Preheat the oven to 400 degrees Fahrenheit.

Combine the almonds, spices, water, coconut milk, coconut oil, 1 teaspoon salt, and cauliflower in a large mixing bowl.

Mix the ingredients well with your hands.

Remove a baking pan from the oven and pour the mixture into it.

Cook for 30 minutes in the oven.

Nutrition

263 calories per serving 4.2 g of fat

4.2% saturated fat

Cholesterol 1,5 micrograms

843 milligrams sodium

12.5 g carbohydrates

2.3 g fiber

Soup with Tortillas and Spring Water

15 minutes are necessary for preparation.

Time to cook: 10 minutes

4 servings

Tortilla soup is a visually pleasing dish made up of a variety of healthy and alkalized foods weaved together to produce a tasty and spicy dinner.

1 ripe avocado (cut into slices); 1 ripe avocado (cut into slices); 1 ripe avocado (cut into slices

1/2 tablespoon coriander 500 milliliters spring water

spinach, 4 handfuls

4 tostadas

Himalayan salt, a pinch

cumin (1 teaspoon)

2 tbsp olive oil (extra virgin)

Instructions:

Cut your tortilla into 5-cm-long, 1-cm-wide strips and toast them gently on a hot grill.

Use spring water to make the veggie broth.

To the broth, add the spinach, cumin, and a touch of salt. Cook for 10 minutes, then remove from the fire and cool.

Serve the soup with tortilla pieces, avocado slices, and extra virgin olive oil on the side.

Nutrition

A serving has 157 calories. 7.2 g of fat

Cholesterol: 2.5 milligrams Saturated fat: 4.8 milligrams

843 milligrams sodium

12.5 g carbohydrates

2.3 g fiber

Soup with a Kick of Minestrone

15 minutes are necessary for preparation.

Time to prepare: 15 minutes

2 servings

The "Hearty Minestrone" is jam-packed with alkaline nutrients and extremely tasty. You are merely doing a wonderful service to your body by preparing it. This vegetable minestrone is rich in minerals and fiber, as well as vitamins and phytonutrients that function as antioxidants.

This dish's combination of carrots, zucchini, and sweet potatoes leaves no doubt that it is delicious, nutritious, and healthy.

Ingredients:

a basil bunch 1 carrot cup sweet potato mashed 1 onion, red

coconut oil, 1 tablespoon 1 cup tomato juice 1 liter vegetable broth cooked beans, 1/2 cup

Chapter 6

Himalayan salt with black pepper

Instructions:

The onion, carrot, and zucchini should all be peeled and diced.

In a big pan, heat the oil for 2 minutes and sauté the onion, carrot, and zucchini.

Combine the tomato juice, stock, and beans in a large mixing bowl.

Bring the mixture to a boil, then add the mashed sweet potato and simmer for 8–10 minutes on low heat.

Add the basil and season with salt and pepper.

Nutrition

Serving size: calorie count: calorie count: calorie count: calorie count: calorie count: 110 6.4 g fat

2.8 g saturated fat 11.3 g carbohydrates

3.5 g fiber

Noodles of Zucchini, served uncooked

15 minutes are necessary for preparation.

Time to cook: 10 minutes

2 servings

3 medium zucchinis, peeled and sliced

spring onions, chopped

Coconut oil is a kind of vegetable oil that is (three tablespoons)

1 coriander bunch (freshly cut) (about 1 tablespoon)

To prepare the sauce, follow these instructions.

a piece of ginger root, grated

a quarter cup of tamari and a quarter cup of tahini

2 tblsp lemon juice or lime juice

Almond butter, 1/4 cup

1 peeled and chopped garlic clove

1 tablespoon sugar (coconut)

Instructions:

Begin by slicing the courgette and carrot noodles very thinly using a mandolin or vegetable peeler.

In a blender, mix the grated ginger, tahini, minced garlic, lime/lemon juice, tamari, almond butter, and coconut sugar to make the sauce.

Blend in a little amount of water until a thick sauce forms.

Finally, toss the zucchini noodles with the sauce in a large mixing bowl.

Before serving, garnish with a squeeze of lime/lemon juice and a sprig of coriander.

Nutrition

229 calories per serving 6.2 g fat

3.8 g saturated fat 5 milligrams of cholesterol

785 milligrams sodium

13.7 g carbohydrate

6.2 g fiber

Quinoa with Spinach Quinoa with Spinach

10 minutes of preparation time is necessary.

Time to prepare: 25 minutes.

4 servings

Ingredients:

cups of freshly chopped fresh spinach cup of cooked quinoa spring water, 1/2 cup

1 finely sliced sweet potato

1 teaspoon coriander powder, ground 1 teaspoon turmeric, 1 tablespoon cumin seeds

1/2 teaspoon ginger (freshly grated) 2 peeled and sliced garlic cloves 1 tablespoon extra-virgin olive oil 1 cup finely chopped onion

1 tablespoon lime juice, freshly squeezed a grain of salt

Instructions:

Cook for 2 minutes with the onion and olive oil in the pan.

Cook for 10 minutes after adding the garlic, ginger, spices, and quinoa.

Cook for another 10 minutes with the spinach, sweet potatoes, and water.

Serve immediately on plates.

Nutrition

268 calories per serving 9.9 g fat

38.8 g carbohydrate 3.4 grams of sugar 7.6 grams of protein

Time to prepare Veggie Soup: 1 hour and 20 minutes

4 person servings

Ingredients:

Cooked Garbanzo Beans (four cups) Pasta (Quinoa) or Pasta (Spelled) (around 4 cups) cooked 4 cups finely chopped mushrooms 3 plum tomatoes, peeled and sliced 1 zucchini, peeled and sliced 2 cups finely chopped butternut squash 1 cup finely chopped red bell pepper 1 red onion, peeled and chopped 2 teaspoons salt Avocado oil (about 2 teaspoons) 2 Tablespoons Basil

Instructions:

Bring a large saucepan halfway full with Spring Water to a boil over high heat.

Getting all of the veggies ready (chop or dice them).

In a large stockpot, combine all ingredients (except the pasta) and spices. Cook for 30 minutes at a low temperature.

5 minutes before the soup is done, stir in the pasta that has been cooked.

Fill a bowl with your Veggie Soup and enjoy!

Tip

As a side dish, serve our Veggie Soup with Tortillas or Spelled Bread.

Nutrition

Serving size: calorie count: calorie count: calorie count: calorie count: calorie count: 210 6.4 g fat

2.8 g saturated fat 11.3 g carbohydrates

3.5 g fiber

Soup made with sourdough

Time to prepare: 1 hour and 20 minutes

4 servings

Ingredients:

Leaves from 4–6 Soursop

2 cups finely chopped kale Quinoa (1 cup)

1 cup chopped Chayote Squash 1 cup finely chopped red bell peppers 1 cup onions, finely diced

1 cup Zucchini, sliced (optional)

1 cup Summer Squash, sliced (optional) 3 tblsp. onion powder

Himalayan Pink Salt, a pinch

1 tablespoon ginger, freshly minced 1 tbsp. oregano leaves, dried

a quarter cup of basil (or parsley)

Instructions:

Make sure all the veggies are ready (chop or dice them).

In a large saucepan, combine all of the ingredients and spices. Add 8 cups of spring water to the mix.

After the mixture reaches a rolling boil, cook it for 30–40 minutes on medium heat.

In a bowl, toss the soup and serve.

Tips

If you don't have Quinoa on hand or don't like for it, rice or handmade pasta may be used instead.

If you don't like spicy cuisine, you may skip the Cayenne Powder in this recipe. You may also serve Sour Soup with Herb Bread instead of Tortillas.

Nutrition

Serving size: calorie count: calorie count: calorie count: calorie count: calorie count: calorie count: 230 6.4 g fat

2.8 g saturated fat 11.3 g carbohydrates 3.5 g fiber

Mushroom Soup is a delicious soup made with mushrooms.

Time to prepare: 3 hours and 20 minutes

4 servings

Ingredients:

3 cups Portobello Mushrooms, 1 cup cooked Garbanzo Beans 2 tbsp. aquafaba (plant-based yoghurt)

1/2 cup red bell peppers, finely chopped kale, finely chopped plum tomatoes butternut squash, chopped

(about 1/2 cup chopped) onions, red, sliced (about half a cup)

2 tsp. Himalayan Pink Salt

2 tblsp. powdered onion (optional) 1 Tablespoon Basil (optional)

1 tsp oregano (oregano) (optional) a smidgeon of ginger powder Grapeseed Oil, 2 tblsp.

Instructions:

In a saucepan, combine all of the ingredients and simmer for 1 hour on low heat. During this time, be sure to stir regularly.

Allow to cool before blending everything together with an immersion blender.

Enjoy the mushroom soup served in bowls!

Tips

If you don't have any prepared Aquafaba on hand, 4 cups spring water may be substituted.

If you don't like spicy cuisine, you may leave out the cayenne powder.

You may serve the Mushroom Soup with Tortillas or Herb Bread as a side dish.

Nutrition

240 calories per serving 2.4 g fat

4.8 g saturated fat 11.3 g carbohydrates 3.5 g fiber

Soup with Garbanzo Beans and Tomatoes

Time to prepare: 1 hour and 20 minutes

4 servings

Ingredients:

Cooked Garbanzo Beans (three cups) 1 finely chopped tomatillo

10 peeled and sliced plum tomatoes 1/2 cup green bell pepper

1/2 cup onions, finely chopped

2 tsp. Himalayan Pink Salt 1 tsp basil powder 1 tsp cayenne pepper powder oregano leaves, 1/2 teaspoon 1/2 teaspoon achiote powder Oil from Grapeseed (about 2 tablespoons) 1 cup of mineral water (optional)

Instructions:

In a large saucepan, combine the tomatillos, onions, bell peppers, grape seed oil, and herbs. On medium heat, sauté veggies for 4–5 minutes, stirring regularly.

Combine the tomatoes, seasonings, Garbanzo Beans, and spring water in a large pot.

On a low heat setting, cook for about 1 hour.

Vegetables should be added to a soup a few minutes before it is completed cooking.

Serve your Spicy Tomato Bean Soup while it's still hot!

Tips

If you want it to be a bit less spicy, use just 1/2 teaspoon of Cayenne pepper. Spicy Tomato Bean Soup may be served with Tortillas or Herb Bread, depending on your desire.

Nutrition

Serving size: calorie count: calorie count: calorie count: calorie count: calorie count: 210 6.4 g fat

2.8 g saturated fat 15.3 g carbohydrate

3.5 g fiber

Gazpacho with Cucumber Cream

Time to prepare: 15 minutes

2 servings

Ingredients

cucumbers

1 avocado (ripe)

a handful of basil, a key lime

Himalayan Pink Salt, a pinch 2 c. fresh spring water

2 tbsp olive oil (extra virgin)

Instructions:

Remove any seeds from the cucumber before peeling it. Using a knife, cut the avocado into pieces.

In a blender, combine all of the ingredients and puree until smooth. Toss in the salt.

Allow 10 minutes for the soup to chill in the refrigerator.

Finish by garnishing the meal with basil leaves, oil, and thinly sliced cucumber.

Enjoy your Cucumber Gazpacho with Cream!

Tips

The Chickpea "Tofu" snack, which is sold separately, works nicely with the Creamy Cucumber Gazpacho.

Nutrition

Serving size: calorie count: calorie count: calorie count: calorie count: calorie count: 135 2.4 g fat

2.4 g saturated fat 11.3 g carbohydrates

3.5 g fiber

Asparagus Soup with Cream

The preparation time is 10 minutes.

Time to prepare: 30 minutes

Ingredients: Ingredients: Ingredients: Ingredients: Ingredients: Ingredients: Ingredients:

2 pound. fresh asparagus, woody stalks removed 2 tablespoons lime juice and 1 lime zest

a quarter cup of coconut milk 1 teaspoon thyme (dried) 1/2 teaspoon oregano, dry

1 head of cauliflower, florets removed 1 tablespoon of minced garlic

1 finely sliced leek

a third of a cup of coconut oil

a smidgeon of Himalayan pink salt

Instructions:

In a large saucepan filled with water, bring the asparagus, leek, and cauliflower to a boil.

In a big saucepan, melt the coconut oil. Combine the cooked veggies, herbs, and lime juice in a mixing bowl. Cook for 5 minutes, stirring occasionally.

Remove the pan from the heat and use an immersion blender to mix everything together.

Allow it cool before serving on plates with lime slices cut on top.

Serve.

Nutrition

Serving size: calorie count: calorie count: calorie count: calorie count: calorie count: 110 6.4 g fat

2.8 g saturated fat 11.3 g carbohydrates

3.5 g fiber

Salad with fruits and vegetables

Time to prepare: 5 minutes

Ingredients: 2 Servings

a cucumber, split in half and sliced

2 cups watercress, torn into bite-sized pieces

2 tablespoons lime juice and 1 lime zest 4 cutlery nuts, peeled and broken into little bits

4 basil leaves, fresh

turmeric powder (1/2 teaspoon)

2 tbsp extra-virgin extra-virgin olive oil Himalayan Pink Salt, a pinch

Instructions:

In a large salad bowl, combine the olive oil and key lime juice. To ensure that they are fully blended, thoroughly mix them together.

Combine the veggies, walnuts, turmeric, lime zest, salt, and herbs in a mixing bowl.

Make sure everything is well combined.

Prepare your Fresh Salad and eat it right now!

Nutrition

Serving size: calorie count: calorie count: calorie count: calorie count: calorie count: calorie count: 92 2.4 g fat

2.4 g saturated fat 11.3 g carbohydrates

6.5 g fiber

Salad du Squash et de Zucchini

Cooking time is 30 minutes + 1 hour in the refrigerator.

Ingredients: 4 servings

2 cups (about 1/2 cup) shredded Zucchini Squash shredded

half a cup of soaking Brazil nuts (overnight or at least 4 hours) 1/4 cup finely chopped Hempseed Milk Onion (about a quarter cup) a quarter teaspoon of dates, coarsely chopped

Himalayan Pink Salt, a pinch lime juice, 2 tablespoons Spring Water (1/2 cup)

Instructions:

In a salad dish, combine all of the thinly sliced veggies.

Blend the dates, hempseed milk, Brazil nuts, lime juice, salt, and 1/2 cup spring water together in a blender. Blend until completely smooth.

Season the veggies with the emulsion that has just been mixed.

Serve right away.

Nutrition

Serving size: calorie count: calorie count: calorie count: calorie count: calorie count: 110 2.6 g fat

2.6 g saturated fat 11.5 g carbohydrates

3.5 g fiber

Salad with mango

Time to prepare: 15 minutes Each serving is 2 oz. Ingredients:

6 tomatoes, plum

mango chunks (1/2 cup) (diced)

the tomatillo (tomatillos are a type of tomato). onions, red (about half a cup diced)

1/4 cup green bell peppers, chopped Cilantro leaves (about half a cup)

Himalayan Pink Salt, a pinch a little amount of onion powder

lime juice, 2 tablespoons

2 tbsp olive oil (extra virgin)

Instructions:

Place all of the veggies in a salad dish and thinly slice them.

Combine the mango, lime juice, and spices in a mixing bowl.

Take pleasure in your Quick Mango Salad!

Tip

You may use our Tortilla Chips as a side dish.

Chapter 7

Chickpea Salad is a salad made with chickpeas

Cooking time is 20 minutes, plus 30–60 minutes in the refrigerator.

Ingredients: 4 servings

2 quarts cooked chickpeas Mayonnaise (about 12 cup vegan)

Roughly chopped red onions (approximately 1/4 cup) 1/2 cup green bell peppers, diced 1 teaspoon dill

a little amount of onion powder

Himalayan Pink Salt, a pinch

Instructions:

Combine chickpeas and vegan mayonnaise in a large mixing basin. Mix.

Combine the other ingredients in a salad dish and toss in the chickpeas. Mix it up a little.

Before serving, chill it for 30–60 minutes.

Serve the Chickpea Salad by tossing everything together.

Nutrition

110 calories per serving 5.4 g fat

1.8 g saturated fat 11.3 g carbohydrates

4.5 g fiber

Salad with "Potatoes" Salad with "Potatoes"

Cooking time is 20 minutes, plus 30 minutes in the refrigerator.

Ingredients: 4 servings

potatoes with a sweet taste

2 courgettes

1 cauliflower

1 cup pre-soaked Brazil Nuts (overnight or at least 4 hours) 1/4 cup green bell peppers, sliced

12 onions

lime juice, 1 tbsp Avocado Oil is a kind of oil that comes from

Himalayan Pink Salt, a pinch Ginger powder, a pinch

spring water, 1/2 cup

CHICKPEA SALAD IS A SALAD MADE WITH CHICKPEAS

Instructions:

1 Combine the Brazil Nuts, Avocado Oil, Lime Juice, seasonings, and 1/2 cup Spring Water in a blender and puree until smooth. After 1 minute of rigorous mixing, you've got a smooth paste. Boil the carrots, sweet potatoes, zucchinis, and onion, then cool and chop them.

Mix everything together in a salad dish.

Allow 30 minutes in the refrigerator to chill before serving.

Plate your "Potato" Salad and serve right away!

Nutrition

274 calories per serving 5.4 g fat

2.8 g saturated fat 19.3 g carbohydrates

4.5 g fiber

Salad with Pickles

Cooking time is 20 minutes, plus 30 minutes in the refrigerator.

2 servings

Ingredients:

1 cup finely sliced cucumbers 12 cup apple cider vinegar, 1/2 cup lime juice 1 tablespoon dill (fresh)

1 teaspoon coriander powder 1 teaspoon Himalayan pink salt

crushed red pepper to taste (or a half teaspoon). Spring Water (1/2 cup)

Instructions:

Using a pestle and mortar, crush the coriander.

In a jar with a tight-fitting lid, combine the cucumber slices, coriander, and the other ingredients. Give it a good shake.

Allow 6–8 hours for it to infuse, stirring it every 1–2 hours during that period.

Serve your Pickle Salad and have pleasure in it.

Nutrition

Serving size: calorie count: calorie count: calorie count: calorie count: calorie count: 110 2.4 g fat

1.4 g saturated fat 16.3 g carbohydrates

3.6 g fiber

Baked Tomato Sauce with Beans

Time to prepare: 1 hour and 40 minutes

4 servings

6 plum tomatoes, peeled and halved

Cooked Garbanzo Beans (three cups)

1/4 cup green bell peppers, sliced Onion, diced (about 1/4 cup)

CHICKPEA SALAD IS A SALAD MADE WITH CHICKPEAS

3 tblsp. Date Syrup

a smidgeonononononononononononononon

Himalayan Pink Salt, a pinch

a slice of ginger that has been freshly grated

a quarter teaspoon powdered turmeric

a quarter teaspoon of powder Cloves

Instructions:

In a blender, combine the Plum Tomatoes, Date Syrup, and herbs until a smooth consistency is achieved.

In a large saucepan, combine the tomato mixture, bell peppers, onions, and Garbanzo Beans.

Cook for 30 minutes over medium heat, tossing occasionally, or until veggies are soft.

Serve.

Nutrition

Serving size: calorie count: calorie count: calorie count: calorie count: calorie count: 110 6.4 g fat

2.8 g saturated fat 11.3 g carbohydrates

3.5 g fiber

Sausage Links Preparation time: 30 minutes

4 servings

Ingredients:

quartered mushrooms (about 1 cup)

cup of garbanzo beans Cooked beans are beans that have been soaked in water and then drained. a half cup onion, finely chopped

4 basil leaves, fresh 1 tblsp. fresh dill

1 tablespoon powdered onion garlic powder, a sprinkle

1 teaspoon sage (dried) (ground) 1 tsp oregano (oregano)

Avocado Oil with a dash of Himalayan Pink Salt (about 2 teaspoons)

Instructions:

Blend all items until smooth (except avocado oil and garbanzo beans).

Blend for another 30 seconds, or until the Garbanzo Beans are fully incorporated into the prepared mixture.

Fill a piping bag halfway with the mixture and snip off a little portion of the bottom corner to make a stencil.

Squeeze the prepared mixture into sausages.

In a pan, heat the avocado oil over medium heat until it is hot.

Cook for 3–4 minutes on each side, or until golden brown on both sides. To prevent their splitting apart, they must be rotated carefully.

Serve with a crisp salad.

Advice

You may eat it with a sauce or a vegan mayonnaise.

476 calories per serving 5.4 g fat

2.8 g saturated fat 16.3 g carbohydrates

3.5 g fiber

DESSERTS

ice cream with chocolate

Time to prepare: 5 minutes

Ingredients: Ingredients: Ingredients: Ingredients: Ingredients: Ingredients: Ingredient

100 g agave nectar

cocoa powder (40 g) 5 g vanilla extract

50 g soy or almond milk cinnamon, a pinch

Instructions:

All of the ingredients, except the cinnamon, should be thoroughly mixed together.

To taste, a pinch of cinnamon.

You may make a nice hot drink by adding extra milk and heating it.

Tiramisu with Pumpkin

Time to prepare: 30 minutes

Ingredients: Ingredients: Ingredients: Ingredients: Ingredients: Ingredients: Ingredient

4 spelt toasts (whole wheat) or 4 spelt cookies (dry)

1 cup pumpkin puree (prepared from steamed pumpkin chunks) 2 tablespoons agave nectar

Soy milk, 4 tblsp 2 gallons of coffee

Cocoa that is sour

Instructions:

Combine the pumpkin, soy milk, and agave syrup in a blender.

Place a single piece of rusks in the bottom of a cup.

Pour the coffee into the mugs.

Cover with pumpkin cream and smooth out evenly.

Unsweetened cocoa powder is sprinkled on top.

Tiramisu', which means "to add life," is a tipicle Italian dessert invented in the mid-nineteenth century in the city of Trevis.

CHICKPEA SALAD IS A SALAD MADE WITH CHICKPEAS

This dish seems to have been devised by a mistress of a pleasure house in order for her to serve it to her patrons. This dessert was deemed aphrodisiac by her.

Salami made with chocolate

Time to prepare: 30 minutes Ingredients: Ingredients: Ingredients: Ingredients: Ingredients: Ingredients: Ingredient

300 grams of dark chocolate with an 85% minimum cocoa content. Rice crackers (150 grams)

Soy milk (200 grams) dried fruit (200 grams)

1 teaspoon powdered cinnamon 1 teaspoon powdered turmeric

Instructions:

Combine the galettes and dried fruit in a food processor.

Microwave the chocolate and set it aside to cool.

Combine the soy milk, cut biscuits, and dried fruit in a mixing bowl.

Combine the ingredients in a mixing bowl and pour onto a baking sheet.

To seal the cylinder, wrap the baking paper in a cylinder and roll up the ends.

Refrigerate the roll for at least two hours.

Unroll the chocolate salami and cut it into pieces.

Deepening: A traditional Italian dessert made particularly after Easter to make use of any remaining Easter egg chocolate.

Beans and chocolate cream

Time to prepare: 30 minutes Ingredients: Ingredients: Ingredients: Ingredients: Ingredients: Ingredients: Ingredient

400 grams black beans, cooked 1/2 cup of your favorite cocoa

Almond milk (three cups)

agave syrup, 1 tablespoon

1 teaspoon powdered cinnamon garnish with sliced strawberries and crumbled dry fruit Preparation:

In a large mixing bowl, combine all ingredients and blend with an immersion blender.

Refrigerate the cream for an hour after dividing it into four glasses.

Serve with strawberry slices as a garnish.

The glycemic index of this dish is modest.

20-minute preparation time for a chocolate and yogurt cake Ingredients: Ingredients: Ingredients: Ingredients: Ingredients: Ingredients: Ingredient

1 jar yoghurt (vegetarian) 125 grams 1 jar sunflower seed oil

agave syrup (half a jar)

1 almond or soy milk jar spelt flour, 1 jar

1 jar rice flour 1 jar rice flour 1 jar rice flour 1 jar rice

1 tbsp cocoa powder, unsweetened 1 baking powder sachet

Preparation:

Fill a large mixing bowl halfway with yogurt.

Mix in all of the remaining ingredients, except the cocoa, until a creamy consistency is achieved.

Divide the dough into two bowls, one of which will contain the bitter cocoa.

Line a cake tin with baking paper and pour the first bowl's dough into it, followed by the second cacao dough in the center.

Preheat oven to 180°F and bake for 25 minutes.

Additional information: This dessert is simple to make because no scales are required!

PLANT BASED DIET MEAL PLAN FOR 14 DAYS

All of the recipes in this book can be used to create your own customized meal plan.

I've created a 14-day meal plan for you below that corresponds to an appropriate period for you to achieve detoxification and activate an anti-inflammatory process in your body.

Feel free to replace some of the dishes in my recipes with others that better suit your tastes.

Or if you are particularly in a hurry you can simplify the daily menu as follows:

for breakfast, prepare a nutritious smoothy with unsweetened vegetable yogurt blended with fresh fruit, half an avocado and a handful of dried fruit

at lunch you can opt for a simple spelled or quinoa salad with lots of fresh vegetables and a fruit\syou can dine with a tasty cereal and mushroom soup combined with a slice spelled bread topped with rosemary and olive oil

the snack can be based on dried fruit or berries.

Please read the valuable rules I have prepared for you before reviewing the 14-Day Meal Plan. The rules will make your cooking time more efficient!

Rules

Before beginning to prepare any meal you should carefully read the daily tips. The snacks are optional.

CHICKPEA SALAD IS A SALAD MADE WITH CHICKPEAS

You can customize your meal by including extras like salads made from fresh vegetables, sauces, fruits, pure agave syrup, tortillas, and so on.

Day 1\sBreakfast: Smoothy with unsweetened vegetable yogurt blended with fresh fruit, half an avocado and agave syrup 4 brazil nuts, ginger tea.

Lunch: Mushroom Soup with Herb Bread lunch A fresh salad with ½ avocado

Dinner: Cabbage Roll Casserole with a Twist Zucchini and Squash Salad.

Snack: Smoothie with avocado and fresh fruit

Preparation Tips:\sMake an extra batch of Mushroom Soup and keep it in the fridge for Day 2

Keep the remaining Herb Bread for Day 2 as a snack

Day 2\sBreakfast: Strawberry Milkshake with vegetable milk A handful of almonds

Lunch: Quinoa with Spinach

Dinner: Gazpacho with Creamy Cucumber A slice of spelled bread with olive oil

Snack: Strawberry Milkshake with vegetable milk Preparation tips:\sMake an additional portion of Quinoa and keep it in the refrigerator for Day 3

Buy two additional portions of spelled bread

Day 3\sBreakfast: Alkaline Porridge with Fruits

A handful of walnuts

Lunch: Pizza with Basil and Olives Lettuce salad with sesame seeds

Dinner: Black bean chili\sTomato and basil salad with olive oil

Snack: Tortilla Chips with a dipping sauce called "Cheese." Preparation tips:

Prepare four extra portions of Black bean chili for Day 5 (look at dinner) (look at dinner).

Prepare a second batch of Tortilla Chips for Day 4 as a backup plan (look at snack) (look at snack).

Day 4\sBreakfast: Coconut Tahini Cookies made with permitted\sflours

A cup of coconut milk

Lunch: Quinoa Burrito Bowl

Thin cut raw courgettes with sesame seeds and avocado oil

Dinner: Pasta with Tomatoes and Spelt

A plate of spinach cooked with avocado oil

Snack: Tortilla Chips with Quick Mango Salsa Preparation tips:\sMake an additional batch of Pasta with Tomatoes and Spelt for Day 5 (look at dinner) (look at dinner).

Preparing an extra portion of Quinoa Burrito Bowl for Day 6 is optional (look at lunch) (look at lunch).

Day 5\sBreakfast: Slice of fresh coconut

A cup of chamomile A little banana

Lunch: Stir-Fry with Zucchini and Broccoli

Dinner: Pasta with Tomatoes and Spelt Cucumber salad with slides of mushrooms and\savocado oil

Snack: A handful of berries and nuts

Preparation tips:\sMake an additional serving of broccoli in the fridge for Day 6. (look at lunch).

1. Preparing an extra portion of Pasta with Tomatoes and Spelt for Day 7 is recommended (look at dinner) (look at dinner).

Breakfast: Raspberry tea\s

Day 6

A slice of spelled bread with thaini butter and agave syrup

A handful of berries

Lunch: Salad de chickpeas\sBroccoli with walnuts and sesame seeds oil

Dinner: Kamut Noodles with Pesto Tomato and basil salad with olive oil

Snack: Strawberry Milkshake with vegetable milk

Preparation tips:

Keep an extra serving of Salad de chickpeas in the refrigerator for Day 8 (look at lunch) (look at lunch).

Keep an extra serving Strawberry Milkshake with vegetable milk for breakfast

Day 7\sBreakfast: Strawberry Milkshake with vegetable milk A handful of walnuts

Lunch: Pasta with Tomatoes and Spelt Zucchini and Squash Salad

Dinner: Links of Sausage\sBroccoli with walnuts and sesame seeds oil

Snack: A handful of almonds

Preparation tips:

Make an extra batch of the Zucchini and Squash Salad or Day 8 (look at lunch) (look at lunch).

Day 8\sBreakfast: Coconut Tahini Cookies made with permitted flours A cup of coconut milk

Lunch: Quinoa Burrito Bowl

Thin cut raw courgettes with sesame seeds and avocado oil

Dinner: Zucchini and Squash Salad\s½ avocado with a slides of tomato and olives

Snacks: Juice from Prickly Pears Preparation tips:

Make an extra batch of Quinoa Burrito Bowl and keep it in the fridge for Day 10. (look at lunch).

Day 9\sBreakfast: Pancakes with Strawberry Jam

Lunch: Okra with a Spicy Twist\sThin cut raw courgettes with sesame seeds and avocado

Dinner: Chickpea Salad\sLettuce salad with sesame seeds

Snack: Strawberry Milkshake with vegetable milk

Preparation tips:

Make an additional batch of Strawberry Milkshake with vegetable milk to use on Day 10 (look at snack) (look at snack).

Preserve an additional serving of Okra with a Spicy Twist for Day 10 (look at lunch) (look at lunch).

Day 10\sBreakfast: Strawberry Milkshake with vegetable milk A handful of almonds

Lunch: Okra with a Spicy Twist\sBroccoli with walnuts and sesame seeds oil

Dinner: Pizza with Basil and Olives Lettuce salad with sesame seeds

Snack: A handful of berries and nuts

Preparation tips:

Day 11 will require an extra portion of Pizza with Basil and Olives (look at dinner) (look at dinner).

Breakfast: Raspberry tea\s

Day 11

A slice of spelled bread with thaini butter and agave syrup

Lunch: Pizza with Basil and Olives Lettuce salad with sesame seeds

Dinner: Zucchini and Squash Salad\s½ avocado with slices of tomato and olives

Snack: Juice from Prickly Pears

Preparation tips:

Keep the leftover Zucchini and Squash Salad for Day 13 in an airtight container (look at dinner) (look at dinner).

Day 12\sBreakfast: Strawberry Milkshake with vegetable milk A handful of walnuts

Lunch: Pasta with Tomatoes and Spelt Zucchini and Squash Salad

Dinner: Links of Sausage

Broccoli with walnuts and sesame seeds oil

Snack: A handful of almonds

Preparation tips:

Reserve a portion of the Pasta with Tomatoes and Spelt for Day 13 of the week (look at lunch) (look at lunch).

Day 13\sBreakfast: Tempeh with Pineapple on the Grill

Lunch: Salad de chickpeas

Broccoli with walnuts and sesame seeds oil

Dinner: Pasta with Tomatoes and Spelt\s½ avocado with slices of tomato and olives Snack: A handful of berries and nuts Preparation tips:\sMaking additional Salad de chickpeas for Day 14 will save you time and money (look at lunch) (look at lunch)

Day 14

Breakfast: Slice of fresh coconut A cup of chamomile

A little banana

Lunch : Green Soup with Alkalizing Properties Tomato and basil salad with olive oil

Dinner: Salad de chickpeas

Cucumber salad with slides of mushrooms and avocado oil

Snacks: A handful of berries and nuts

CPSIA information can be obtained
at www.ICGtesting.com
Printed in the USA
LVHW061328070422
715596LV00006B/128

9 781804 386156